THE
VITAMIN
CURE
for Diabetes

IAN E. BRIGHTHOPE, M.D.

ANDREW W. SAUL, PH.D.,
SERIES EDITOR

Basic
Health
PUBLICATIONS, INC.

The information contained in this book is based upon the research and personal and professional experiences of the authors. It is not intended as a substitute for consulting with your physician or other healthcare provider. Any attempt to diagnose and treat an illness should be done under the direction of a healthcare professional.

The publisher does not advocate the use of any particular healthcare protocol but believes the information in this book should be available to the public. The publisher and authors are not responsible for any adverse effects or consequences resulting from the use of the suggestions, preparations, or procedures discussed in this book. Should the reader have any questions concerning the appropriateness of any procedures or preparation mentioned, the authors and the publisher strongly suggest consulting a professional healthcare advisor.

Basic Health Publications, Inc.
www.basichealthpub.com

Library of Congress Cataloging-in-Publication Data
is on file with the Library of Congress

ISBN-13: 978-1-59120-290-5 (Pbk.)

Editing: Margaret Moran and Andrew W. Saul
Typesetting/Book design: Gary A. Rosenberg
Cover design: Mike Stromberg

ISBN-13: 978-1-68162-827-1 (Hardcover)

CONTENTS

Dedicated to My Mum,
Moya

If we could give the right amount of nourishment and exercise, not too little and not too much, we would have found the safest way to health.

—HIPPOCRATES

ACKNOWLEDGEMENTS

I would like to thank the following people who supported me while writing this book or provided some of the many references: my PA, Susanne Powell; David Kirk; Charithra Attanayake; David Doolan; George Panagios; Senator Guy Barnett; Andrew W. Saul; Dr. Damien Downing; and all my staff. My special thanks to my wife Jill and our two adult children, Sarah-Jane and Daniel.

FOREWORD

Professor Ian Brighthope is a pioneer in nutritional and environmental medicine. He's also a strong-minded Aussie, which is just as well considering all the heat he has had to take over the years. It's no surprise that he studied agriculture before medicine—vets are way ahead of doctors in understanding the importance of nutrition, and farmers have known about it for millennia: finding the good pastures, the clean water for their animals. How did we manage to forget all that in relation to ourselves? I am thankful for doctors like Ian, who are able to see through the disinformation and ground us anew as humans who need good food and a safe planet to live on.

It is shameful that so many attacks have been made on Ian by the medical profession; he has had to become an expert in dealing with them. One reason that he (nearly always) succeeds is that he is (nearly always) right about medicine. Of course that's also a reason why he has been attacked; vested interests never want to hear the truth if it threatens profits or power.

Ian knows his stuff and he learns from his patients. This makes him an ideal person to explain to you about diabetes and how to deal with it. Some of the facts in this book are the old fundamentals that we managed somehow to forget. Many of the insights are right up-to-the-minute scientific news. Sometimes the two combine to complete the circle. Didn't your Granny go on about the importance of a good night's sleep, for instance? Scientists have finally caught up with her, and started to describe how lack of sleep disrupts your hormones, and can actually put weight on you. Obesity, the Metabolic Syndrome and diabetes are turning into the biggest killers around; but when you rethink and remodel your life and your diet, believe me, the benefits can be amazing.

When you turn over this page, one of the first things this book will tell you is that more than 220 million people worldwide have diabetes. If they all bought this book that would make the author a multi-millionaire! It won't happen, of course. But if you or someone you care about is one of that 220 million, you're holding in your hands a potentially life-saving opportunity to change that. One that doesn't depend on potentially dangerous drugs; one that tackles the fundamentals—the food we eat, the sunlight on our skin, the worries that keep us awake nights—and offers real solutions, based on lifestyle changes and safe, natural therapies.

This book doesn't lie to you. This isn't one of those internet "send $40 for our miracle cure" promos. Dr. Brighthope isn't suggesting you can just walk away from your doctor and do it all by yourself. Diabetes can be a killer. All the more reason to do everything you can, and not to rely on your prescriptions alone. You really can take back control of your own life and health; this book will tell you how.

Damien Downing, M.D.
London, UK

INTRODUCTION

We have an epidemic of obesity and diabetes in Western industrialized nations. The industrial revolution has changed the world and our lives, forever. There have been many developments to our advantage such as the automobile, railroad, airplane, better homes and an abundance of food for many nations. Food processing is going to be our downfall unless we do something about it. The most sinister separation has been the removal of sugar from sugar cane and sugar beet. It would take a very long time chewing on sugar cane to extract a teaspoon of sugar, yet a machine can do it very effectively and provide literally buckets of sugar for each of us to consume every year. Nearly every processed food contains this potentially deadly poison. It's so easy to drink a can of soda—it's not so easy to accept that one can contains over ten teaspoons of sugar, most of which is stored in the body as fat.

I remember attending two international congresses on obesity in the 1980s at which not one speaker discussed the harmful effects of sugar. When I questioned the relationship of sugar to human diseases, a professor of nutrition and medicine replied that there was no medical evidence that sugar caused obesity, diabetes, or heart disease.

Those congresses were sponsored by the soft drink manufacturers, the ice-cream manufacturers, the sugar industry and the dietician's association whose journal was also sponsored by the

1

sugar industry interests. Diabetes, sometimes called "the sugar disease," is not always caused by sugar, but sugar plays a major role in most cases. As you will see, there are many other factors that contribute to diabetes. I hope you enjoy this book and if you are diabetic, that it assists you in your journey to better health. If you are not a diabetic, I hope that it gives you some direction in assisting a loved one with the disease. I took this journey with my mother after she was diagnosed with diabetes in 1968; a time when there was much less information than there is today.

The next time you enjoy a soft drink, ice cream, cake, or another sugary treat, please remember that these foods are converted to blood sugar that is deposited directly into fat cells if it is not used for energy. The sugar in your soft drink is called *sucrose*—commonly known as table sugar—and it consists of two simpler sugars: glucose, which becomes blood sugar, and fructose, also known as "fruit sugar" because it is the same sugar in fruits and honey. Just as the glucose that is not used for energy is stored as fat, fructose also goes directly into fat cells as triglycerides and fatty acids.

The shame and pity of all of this is that most people who enjoy these sugar-laden products do not realize that every mouthful they take is making them fat, little by little. I feel so sad when I see parents and children pouring this garbage down their throats—garbage that nutritionists still say is a part of a healthy diet. Yes, I am deliberately being provocative here, but that is because all the other reasonable strategies to change have failed.

In January 2011, the medical journal *Circulation* published an article that linked high added sugar intake to increased risk of heart and blood vessel disease in adolescents in the United States. At last, the published science is catching up with the nutritional and orthomolecular doctors who have been making scientifically based claims about the harmful effects of sugar for decades, including the fact that there is an increased risk of cardiovascular disease among adults who eat a high-carbohydrate, high-sugar diet. In the *Circulation* report, the average daily intake of added sugars was found to be about 22 percent of the total energy intake of an adolescent—a rather frightening figure that reflects over-consumption of calorie-dense, nutrient-poor foods. Further, the more sugar adolescents consumed, the lower their blood levels of the "good" (high-density lipoprotein, HDL) cholesterol that protects against heart disease. Basically, sugar is pushing out the molecules that protect against heart attacks. Added sugar also increased "bad" fats in the blood, including triglycerides and low-density lipoprotein (LDL) cholesterol. For adolescents who were overweight or obese, the added sugars were connected to insulin resistance. To sum it up, these young people are already well on their way to developing metabolic syndrome and diabetes.

These findings make me both angry and disappointed. I am disappointed in our health care system and medical practitioners who continue to ignore the importance of sugar in disease, and I am angry with our governments and the sugar industry—both of which continue to allow huge quantities of this energy-rich, nutrient-poor substance to be added to foods. Sugar is a dangerous chemical. We have easily become addicted to it, and it is slowly killing us. It causes physical illness, psychiatric disease, learning and behavior disorders, and perhaps even crime. Clearly it is a precursor to other, more addictive, substances such as tobacco, alcohol, and drugs—all of which negatively affect physical and mental health.

Unfortunately, sugar is ubiquitous. It is everywhere in nearly everything we consume, stealthily infiltrating our body systems and slowly but surely destroying molecules, cells, and tissues. Remember how long it took for the authorities to recognize and acknowledge the damaging effects on our health caused by tobacco? Alcohol causes more psychiatric and physical disease than tobacco and is associated with a massive amount of trauma and crime. It is a greater evil than tobacco. To relegate alcohol

to the current status of tobacco products is going to take generations. To convince the consumer and governments of the harmful effects of sugar will take even longer, which leads me
to believe that our disease orientated health care systems will
bear the burden of sugar- and alcohol-fueled diseases for many
generations.

PART 1

UNDERSTANDING DIABETES

CHAPTER 1

WHAT IS DIABETES?

Man is a food-dependent creature. If you don't feed him,
he will die. If you feed him improperly, part of him will die.
—EMANUEL CHERASKIN, M.D., D.M.D.

Diabetes mellitus is a chronic illness that affects the way the body uses food for energy. It is characterized by high blood levels of a sugar called *glucose,* which is the main source of fuel for the body. In diabetes, the body is not able to effectively use glucose to fuel its needs, leaving cells starved for energy.

During digestion, food is broken down into components that can be absorbed and used by the body in all of its daily functions. Most of the food we eat is broken down into glucose, which is released into the bloodstream as food is digested, so that it can be used for energy. The corresponding rise in blood glucose levels after a meal stimulates a gland called the pancreas, located behind the stomach, to release insulin. Insulin is a hormone that helps move glucose from the bloodstream into muscle, fat, and liver cells. With the assistance of other factors, including the glucose tolerance factor (GTF), insulin opens up channels in the cell membrane that allow glucose molecules to enter the cell to produce energy.

In people who have diabetes, the pancreas either produces little or no insulin, or the body's cells do not respond well to the

DIABETES STATISTICS

- Worldwide, more than 220 million people have diabetes.

- In 2004, an estimated 3.4 million people died from the consequences of high blood sugar.

- More than 80% of diabetes deaths occur in low- and middle-income countries.

- WHO projects that diabetes deaths will double between 2005 and 2030.

insulin that is produced. As a result, glucose is unable to enter into the cells and instead builds up in the blood, where it is useless as a fuel source and dangerous to the body as well. Some of the glucose also spills over into the urine and passes out of the body during urination.

As we will discuss in the next section, there are several types of diabetes, and multiple reasons why people may develop the disease. However, the signs and symptoms are largely the same. These include:

- Fatigue

- Sugar cravings

- Psychological changes

- Frequent urination (polyuria)

- Excessive thirst (polydipsia)

- Excessive hunger

- Unexplained weight loss

- Poor wound healing

Chronically high blood sugar levels become toxic to many of the tissues and organs of the body. Over time, uncontrolled high blood sugar levels can affect almost every part of the body, causing complications including blindness, kidney failure, brain and nerve damage, heart disease, and atherosclerosis.

TYPES OF DIABETES

There are three main types of diabetes. In type 1 diabetes, the pancreas produces little or no insulin, and daily insulin injections are required to compensate for this lack. By contrast, in type 2 diabetes, the pancreas does make some insulin, but it is not enough to keep blood glucose levels within a normal range, typically because the body's cells do not respond well to insulin. Gestational diabetes develops during pregnancy in women who did not previously have diabetes before becoming pregnant. Although this form of diabetes may resolve itself after the child is born, a woman who has gestational diabetes is at higher risk of developing type 2 diabetes later in life.

In addition to the three major types of diabetes outlined above, we will also discuss two other forms of the disease here. Individuals who have type 1.5 diabetes, also known as latent autoimmune diabetes in adults (LADA), at first do not require daily insulin injections because the pancreas still produces some insulin. However, over time, the ability of the pancreas to make insulin declines until insulin injections are necessary to compensate for the lack. There is also a type of diabetes known as secondary diabetes, in which diabetes is a secondary condition that results from another illness (for example, a condition that impairs or damages the pancreas).

Let's now take a closer look at the similarities and differences among the different types of diabetes.

Type 1 Diabetes

Although type 1 diabetes can affect anyone of any age, it has often been called juvenile diabetes and childhood onset diabetes because it is more typically diagnosed in children, adolescents, and young adults. It is also known as insulin-dependent diabetes (IDDM) because daily insulin injections are necessary for a person with type 1 diabetes to survive.

Type 1 diabetes occurs when the body's own immune system attacks cells in the pancreas called beta cells, which are responsible for producing insulin. When the beta cells are destroyed, the pancreas is unable to make the insulin required to help cells take up glucose from the blood for fuel. One of the concerns in type 1 diabetes is that, in the absence of sufficient glucose, the body begins to burn fat for energy. The breakdown of fat produces ketones, acids that are highly toxic, particularly to the nervous system. When ketones build up in the blood and the brain, a condition known as diabetic ketoacidosis (DKA) can result. Without immediate treatment, DKA can cause the body to shut down, eventually leading to coma and even death.

Because the function of the immune system is to fight off foreign invaders such as viruses and bacteria, we do not fully understand why this defense turns against the body it's meant to protect and attacks the beta-cells. However, there is evidence that a great number of factors may play a role in this mutiny. These include diet, food allergies or intolerances, chemicals, antibiotics, gut bacteria, infections, vitamin and mineral deficiencies, and possibly the failure of the immune system to be properly stimulated by typical childhood infections such as measles, mumps, and German measles.

Type 2 Diabetes

Type 2 diabetes is the most common form of the disease, affecting 80 percent of people with diabetes. This type of diabetes has been known as adult-onset diabetes, due to the fact it is more often diagnosed in people who are middle-aged or older. It is also called non-insulin dependent diabetes (NIDDM), because individuals who have this form of the disease do not necessarily require daily insulin injections as long as their illness is well controlled through other measures.

Type 2 diabetes is a disorder of sugar metabolism. Unlike in type 1 diabetes, the pancreas still does make some insulin. However, either the amount of insulin that is produced is less than what is required to normalize blood sugar levels, or the body's cells are not able to effectively use the insulin that is produced, due to a condition known as *insulin resistance*. As mentioned above, insulin attaches to receptors on the cell membrane in order to open channels that allow glucose molecules to pass through. In people who have type 2 diabetes, too little insulin in combination with too many nonfunctioning insulin receptors means that glucose is not able to enter the body's cells, and instead remains in the bloodstream or passes out of the body through the urine.

Despite the name "non-insulin dependent diabetes," type 2 diabetes is a very serious condition with extremely serious complications. Although individuals with type 2 diabetes may not initially require insulin injections, about a third of all patients who have this form of the disease will eventually need daily insulin injections if they survive fifteen years with the disease. Unfortunately, insulin injections can actually cause further damage. Insulin actually stimulates deposition of cholesterol fatty blobs on the inside of the arteries, and this results in poor blood flow to vital organs such as the brain, heart, liver, kidneys, and legs. Poor circulation, in turn, can lead to tissue death, or gangrene, in the feet and legs, which may require amputation. Blockages can be fatal if they are the cause of a heart attack or stroke.

Although anyone can develop type 2 diabetes, some people are at higher risk, including those who are obese or overweight, women who have had gestational diabetes, people with type 2 diabetes in their family, individuals who have metabolic syndrome (discussed later), people who smoke, and those who have a sedentary lifestyle. Unfortunately, type 2 diabetes may exist for many years before it is detected, and complications such as cardiovascular disease, eye disease, and kidney disease may be well established even before they are diagnosed.

Of the risk factors listed above, of the biggest problems our society faces is obesity. It is a consequence of our lifestyle—we're taking in more calories than our bodies need or can use. We have ignored this dilemma for too long, and it is essentially a time bomb that has the potential to bankrupt even a healthy economy. Public health authorities have acknowledged this possibility. In my opinion, the sugar industry should bear the brunt of the blame for the current obesity epidemic, and the alcohol and fast fat foods industries are tied for second place. The relationship of refined carbohydrates—including sugar, white flour, and alcohol—to obesity and its related diseases is akin to the link we have seen between tobacco and lung cancer. In fact, when we compare the effects of tobacco and sugar, we can see that sugar intake has done more than tobacco use. And that is saying something.

Obese and overweight people are more prone to diabetes and, without exception, will be major health liabilities into the future to both themselves and their loved ones unless they trim down. The good news is, people with type 2 diabetes can avoid having to take insulin injections by making important lifestyle changes, including changing diet and adopting a regular exercise program.

Gestational Diabetes

Gestational diabetes sometimes develops during pregnancy in women who did not previously have diabetes before becoming pregnant. Up to 5 percent of pregnant women develop this form of diabetes. Although gestational diabetes may disappear after the child is born, a woman who has been diagnosed with this type is at higher risk of developing type 2 diabetes later in life, particularly if she has other risk factors, including a poor diet (high in sugar, refined carbohydrates, and alcohol), obesity, and sedentary lifestyle. In fact, between a quarter and a half of women who have had gestational diabetes will eventually develop type 2 diabetes. Of course, this is preventable by eating a healthy diet, maintaining normal body weight, exercising, and taking nutritional supplements to maintain optimal health, correct deficiencies, and improve pancreatic and genetic function.

If gestational diabetes is not well controlled during a woman's pregnancy, high blood sugar can affect the developing baby, causing birth defects to the brain and heart, skeletal and muscular malformations, and increased risk of miscarriage. Uncontrolled high blood sugar can cause the baby to grow very large with a higher than average birth weight, which can complicate labor and delivery. Additionally, because the mother passes on high quantities of glucose through her blood, the baby's pancreas must produce a great deal more insulin than is normal in an attempt to counteract toxic blood sugar levels. Overproduction of insulin and chronic high blood sugar can impede the baby's lung development, resulting in acute respiratory distress and lung failure at birth. If fetal distress (stress of the baby's heart and lungs) is detected and a caesarean section recommended, in addition to the prescribed treatment and lung support for the baby, I would highly recommend the use of intravenous vitamin C for the mother and baby and intravenous glutathione—a very useful antioxidant—to reduce the oxidative damage to both caused by the diabetes, the surgery, and the oxygen given to the newborn.

Unfortunately, the incidence of gestational diabetes is on the rise, nearly doubling every five years. This contributes to the explosive increase in health-care funding. A woman who is overweight when she becomes pregnant has a greater chance of developing gestational diabetes, and having a baby with many problems at birth and then it growing up with a much greater chance of being obese and developing diabetes also. However, while these trends may be in the genes, a healthy lifestyle can prevent the unhealthy expression of these genes.

Type 1.5 Diabetes

About 20 percent of people who are diagnosed with type 2 diabetes actually have a condition called type 1.5 diabetes, also known as slow onset type 1 diabetes or latent autoimmune diabetes in adults (LADA). People who have type 1.5 diabetes are usually not overweight, have little or no resistance to insulin, and do not initially require insulin injections for treatment. They often do not have other risk factors of type 2 diabetes, such as high blood pressure and high triglycerides. However, because type 1.5 diabetes is often misdiagnosed as type 2 diabetes, the course of treatment at the beginning includes making dietary changes, starting a program of regular exercise, and taking medications prescribed for type 2 diabetes.

Individuals who have type 1.5 diabetes will at first respond well to the treatment program because their bodies are still able to produces insulin. Yet, over time, these measures become less effective. This is because type 1.5 diabetes is similar to type 1 diabetes in that it is an autoimmune disease. In other words, the body's immune system attacks its own tissues—in this case, the pancreas. It may be possible, in the early stages of the disease, to influence the immune system in a positive manner by undertaking an elimination diet, removing foods from the diet that might be causing the body to have an autoimmune response. Foods that should be considered eliminating from the diet include wheat and other gluten containing grains, dairy foods, yeast and any other food showing positive on an IgG test. While there is no absolute certainty in this approach, for those who are willing, an elimination diet may require discipline but it can also produce dividends in terms of better health. Nutritional supplements and the herb Portulaca are very helpful and may stave off the need for insulin.

Secondary Diabetes

As the name suggests, secondary diabetes occurs as a result of some other disease that causes chronically elevated blood glucose levels. In other words, diabetes is not the main, but it is caused, in some way, by the main illness. A wide range of health problems, and a number of medications, can damage the pancreas, including:

- Poisoning by alcohol abuse.

- Cystic fibrosis, which causes cysts to form in the pancreas.

- Pancreatic cancer, particularly aggressive adenocarcinomas in the cells that line the pancreas.

- Cushing's disease, which results from prolonged exposure of the body's tissues to high levels of the hormone cortisol produced by the adrenal glands. Excessive use of cortisone or similar steroid hormones to treat conditions such as asthma, lupus, rheumatoid arthritis, and others can also cause high blood sugar.

- Acromegaly, a rare hormone disorder caused by overproduction of growth hormone by the pituitary gland, usually due to a tumor. Symptoms of this condition include enlarged feet, hands, and facial bones; decreased muscle strength and fatigue; and high blood glucose levels. Growth hormone is sometimes taken as a part of an anti-aging program and this could result in diabetes if the doses are too high.

- Hemochromatosis, a genetic disorder in which the body absorbs too much iron from the gastrointestinal tract. The excess iron builds up in the cells of the liver, heart, pancreas, and other organs, damaging and eventually destroying them.

- Medications, including many common antibiotics, anti-inflammatory drugs and painkillers, cholesterol-lowering drugs, antidepressants and tranquilizers, treatments for heart and stomach problems, and—perhaps most surprising—even medications used to control blood sugar levels in type 2 diabetes.

- Diuretics, which flush salt and fluids from the body. Chronic use of these substances can cause high blood sugar, referred to by the medical profession as idiopathic hyperglycemia (high blood glucose due to an unknown cause). If doctors were properly trained in nutritional biochemistry, they would appreciate the importance of minerals such as zinc, chromium and

MOYA: A TRUE STORY

Moya was a very special person. In 1968 her entire system nearly broke down when she was diagnosed with thyrotoxicosis (too much thyroid hormone). She had lost about 45 pounds in weight in a very short period of time and had been admitted to the hospital in a coma. She had been acutely ill and nearly died. The coma had been caused by ketoacidosis (excessive accumulation of the byproducts of fat breakdown, called ketones). The ketoacidosis resulted from a severe case of diabetes occurring at the same time as the thyrotoxicosis. The management of her condition in the hospital was excellent and she was discharged reasonably well after having radioactive iodine treatment to the thyroid gland and injecting 86 units of insulin per day for the diabetes. A little while later she was also diagnosed with pernicious anemia, a condition in which vitamin B_{12} is not absorbed into the body because of a breakdown in the stomach caused by autoimmune disease. She required regular vitamin B_{12} injections to correct this deficiency and these injections were for life.

Moya had a number of diseases in different systems of the body. In fact her immune system had essentially broken down. Once the diabetes had come under control she started to gain weight and in fact quite a lot of weight. The very high doses of insulin that she needed to keep her blood sugar under control also caused repeated attacks of hypoglycemia, or low blood sugar. These attacks required the use of intravenous glucose. One could say that her diabetes was very poorly controlled and the dieticians at the time had placed her on sugary biscuits and refined carbohydrates that made her sugar swings even worse. This went on for many years during which time she developed hypercholesterolemia and atherosclerosis from the insulin injections. Eventually this lead to heart disease and disease of the arteries to the legs and feet. She was always tired and found it difficult to function but she loved to get out into the garden.

In 1974, her son graduated from medical school and decided to change her diet and give her some vitamins and minerals, which he believed from the available literature at the time may be of benefit to her. These were simply high doses of vitamin B complex, vitamin C, Vitamin E, zinc and magnesium. She was later given some extra vitamin B_6 and with this program over the next three to six months her energy levels improved, she lost weight and her insulin requirements were dropped from 86 units per day to 26 units per day. The heart failure that she had experienced improved and her capacity for exercise and gardening dramatically improved. However, the damage from the high doses of insulin for many years had taken its toll and caused the deposition of cholesterol in her arteries.

The major problem was the arteries to the legs and feet. The vascular surgeon in 1978 was forced to perform bypass surgery to take blood from the arteries in the pelvis to the arteries in the lower legs because Moya's feet had turned cold, blue, and had no pulses. Another series of operations later resulted in bypasses from the arteries in the armpit taking blood to the arteries in the pelvis. Thank goodness that her diet and supplement regime by that time had her diabetes and metabolic syndrome under control. She was fit enough despite all the vascular disease to undergo the surgeries.

Moya managed very well for a year or two until her son arrived home from an overseas conference and discovered that the tips of three of the toes on the left foot had turned black—a sign that gangrene had developed. The vascular surgeon advised immediate amputation of her leg. This news was devastating for a lady who had fought so hard all of these years to overcome the pain and suffering of a number of chronic degenerative diseases.

Her son was aware of a treatment called chelation therapy being conducted in New Zealand and the United States that improved blood flow in patients with atherosclerosis. He contacted his colleagues in New Zealand, who advised him about the protocols of chelation therapy. In short, chelation therapy is the intravenous administration of a substance called EDTA (ethylenediaminetetraacetic acid; you can see why we abbreviate it!) with magnesium and a mixture of other vitamins and minerals. Her son admitted her to a private hospital in Melbourne, Australia, for six weeks and administered the EDTA chelation therapy twice a week. After three weeks of treatment, Moya's feet had turned pink and were pain-free. Scabs had formed at the tips of two of her black toes and her well-being had improved immensely. Her mind was sharper than ever and her sense of humor returned. Another three weeks passed and new tissue had formed at the tips of two toes. The scabs had fallen off. Only the tip of one toe remained blackened.

After her discharge from hospital, Moya returned to the vascular surgeon who removed the tip of that single toe and left her leg intact. He did not ask about how the other toes had healed. Moya had another eight years of reasonably good health and passed away in 1988 following a massive heart attack.

This case history is especially poignant for me. I am the son mentioned above. Moya was my mother.

magnesium in the control of blood glucose levels. It is these very minerals that are washed out of the body by the diuretic drugs that are used to remove excess salt and water.

- Low levels of the male hormone testosterone, which may be responsible for the failure of insulin to stimulate its receptors. This is an example of the lack of a hormone aggravating diabetes, which can also have a negative effect on a man's sex life.

When it is possible to treat the primary illness, secondary diabetes may resolve itself once the body's systems are returned to balance.

METABOLIC SYNDROME AND DIABETES

Metabolic syndrome, once called "syndrome X," is a cluster of conditions that occur together and increase the risk of disease, such as diabetes, cardiovascular disease (heart attack and stroke), and cancer. These risk factors can be grouped together into what is sometimes referred to as the "deadly quartet": high blood pressure; insulin resistance; excess body fat, particularly around the waist; and abnormal cholesterol levels—high "bad" LDL cholesterol, low "good" HDL cholesterol—in combination with high triglycerides. Although having just one of these conditions doesn't warrant a diagnosis of metabolic syndrome in and of itself, it does indicate a risk of disease. This risk increases with the number of risk factors an individual shows. However, aggressive lifestyle changes can delay or even prevent the development of serious health problems.

What Is Metabolic Syndrome?

There's more to body fat than meets the eye, and not all fat functions in the same way. Important distinctions need to be made among the different types of fat we carry. Once considered an "inert energy storage depot," fatty tissue is now recognized as a critical hormone-producing organ. This gives us a unique understanding of the way metabolic syndrome affects the body. It also means that by changing body fat distribution, we can reduce insulin resistance, sugar intolerance, and high levels of blood fats such as cholesterol and triglycerides. Even modest reductions in the fat that accumulates around the waist can reverse metabolic syndrome and reduce the risk of diabetes and other serious illnesses.

From watching television programs, it is easy to assume that fat is just an unsightly accumulation of excess body mass. On the other hand, it is also easy to assume that just because you are overweight or obese you are a candidate for metabolic syndrome and its deadly consequences. In fact, some obese individuals are quite healthy and demonstrate none of the conditions that characterize metabolic syndrome. This phenomenon is also seen in certain ethnic groups, such as Micronesian Nauruans, Melanesians, and Indian-Fijians. Without a doubt, the most extreme example would have to be Japanese Sumo wrestlers. Despite being obviously extremely obese, these individuals are nonetheless extremely fit and healthy—they are athletes after all. They are the "fit and fat." These people fall into a category of the metabolically normal obese (MNO). But here's the rub: after they retire from the sport and discontinue their rigorous training, Sumo wrestlers then develop insulin resistance and metabolic syndrome.

How does this variance come about? The simple answer is that Sumo wrestlers have a large percentage of their body fat stores as subcutaneous adipose tissue (SCAT). *Subcutaneous* means "just under the skin" and *adipose tissue* means "fat"—so SCAT is fat just under the skin. As far it relates to metabolic syndrome, SCAT accumulation is not the type of fat that increases the risk of metabolic syndrome and its associated diseases. Rather, it is the accumulation of visceral adipose tissue (VAT) that plays a critical role in the development of metabolic syndrome. *Visceral* refers to the deep internal organs inside the abdomen such as the intestines, liver, and kidneys, so VAT is fat that is buried deep inside the abdomen surrounding the intestines.

On the flip side of the Sumo equation, you have individuals whose weight appears normal, yet they have metabolic syndrome, usually because they have high levels of VAT. This supports the idea that conditions such as insulin resistance—and, therefore, its effects on glucose being taken up by cells—have more to do with where the fat is located rather than the total amount of body fat. Fat that accumulates in the abdominal region is comprised of both SCAT and VAT. In general, VAT accounts for up to 20 percent of total fat in men and 5 to 8 percent in women.

Adipose tissue was once considered an inactive storage depot, but it actually shows a great deal of metabolic activity. In fact, it is very much like a major fireworks display on New Years Eve that never stops and does not, on the surface, appear to be doing too much damage. However, we now know that fat is continuously being stored in and released from adipose tissue. Insulin isn't responsible only for moving glucose into muscle cells—it also promotes glucose uptake into fat cells. Once glucose enters fat cells, it can be converted to glycerol or fatty acids, which together form triglycerides. Thus, fat cells affect triglyceride and free fatty acid levels, which explains in part why central obesity is a risk factor for other conditions.

You could say that abdominal VAT results in a kind of metabolic disharmony, disrupting chemical messengers and signaling systems that regulate appetite, energy balance, and fat storage. Adipose tissue is also now recognized as an active endocrine gland that secretes several peptide hormones. One of these hormones, leptin, plays a role in appetite and metabolism. Another hormone, resistin, appears to be linked to insulin resistance. Adipose tissue also releases chemical messengers called *cytokines* that interact with immune cells. Cytokines called TNF-alpha and interleukin 6T cause low-grade inflammation and can damage the lining of the arteries. The release of these and other chemicals from adipose tissue explains in part why central obesity is a marker of impaired glucose tolerance and a risk factor for cardiovascular disease. Unfortunately, the ongoing dynamic balance these chemicals initiate is tilted unfavorably in the direction of continuing fat storage and inflammation.

The downstream affects of stress and worry are also associated with an increased abdominal girth—the VAT belly. Chronic stress increases the hormone cortisol; it also increases VAT in abdominal tissue. Repeated episodes of stress that stimulate cortisol secretion from the adrenal glands can eventually damage the part of the brain (hippocampus) that slows down the production of cortisol. This might play a role in VAT accumulation.

A very dangerous situation arises in the VAT belly. The fat

TYPE 2 INSULIN DEPENDENT DIABETES: A CASE HISTORY

Bill was an extremely busy executive in the real estate industry who had been under stress for many years. Two years prior to seeing me he had been diagnosed with type 2 diabetes and unsuccessfully treated with diet and drugs. His diabetic specialist prescribed for him 30 units of insulin per day by injection in the morning and at night. His diet was inadequate and he continued to drink between 2 to 4 standard drinks of different alcoholic beverages every day. He suffered from tiredness, irritability and following the insulin injections had gained weight and his cholesterol and triglycerides had gone through the roof. He said that he had still at least 10 good years of productive work in front of him but was unable to visualize himself achieving anything with his current state of health. He was motivated to make some lifestyle changes and we worked together with his wife to ensure that his passage into and through his management program would be smooth and effective. Bill started walking twice a day in the morning and at night. He changed his complex carbohydrate diet to a diet in which he ate small protein rich snacks throughout the day. He had a family history of diabetes and autoimmune disease and tests revealed that he had antibodies to wheat and wheat gluten and to the enzymes involved in celiac disease. Therefore it was logical for him to go onto a gluten free diet. He stopped his alcohol and took up meditation.

As would be expected in someone with gluten sensitivity, Bill had a number of nutritional deficiencies and imbalances. These were corrected and it wasn't long before we were able to reduce his insulin to 20 units per day and within three months he was on 10 units per day and extremely well controlled. His diabetic specialist conceded that he no longer needed the insulin. I followed Bill up for another 15 years during which time he had no requirements for insulin or diabetic drugs. He stayed on a program of nutritional supplements including vitamin C complex, vitamin E complex, a high-dose B complex, high-dose niacin, high-dose vitamin B_6, zinc, chromium, magnesium, and some herbal medicines. His cholesterol and triglycerides return to normal and his abnormal liver function caused by the alcohol intake also returned to normal.

With this program his cravings for sweets, sugar and alcohol all disappeared and his comments to me were that he had never felt so well in all his life and was achieving more in his occupation and profession than he had in his 30s.

There is an important lesson in this case. It is that by the re-establishment of the normal building blocks of nutrition, addictions and cravings can be cured, some medications can be stopped including some life-saving medications, physical and mental well-being can be improved and individual functionality and achievement may be maximized. Scientific and medical researchers should take note of cases like this. Bill's genes had been abused by his lifestyle. He was motivated to change, fed his genes right, and they responded with the reward of well-being. This life change is available to everyone.

cells deep inside the abdomen can actually take the used breakdown parts of old cortisol molecules and recreate more cortisol. This creates a local cycle that promotes the production of more cortisol and therefore more central adiposity (VAT belly) and more insulin resistance. The Metabolic Syndrome can be self-perpetuating.

In chronic stress, elevated cortisol levels also cause an increase in blood pressure, while at the same time having a negative effect on arterial blood flow. There are even studies that show that episodes of mental stress can have a negative affect on circulation, constricting blood vessels even in young healthy people. Psychological stress can also reduce the clearance of triglycerides and disturb hormones that help regulate appetite and energy storage such as leptin.

Meditation plays an equally important role in weight management as does exercise.

Factors such as sleep debt and chronic stress levels should also be taken into account. All of these can influence the way the body stores and utilizes energy. In order to mobilize abdominal fat it is extremely important that we mount a simultaneous, multiple therapeutic attack on a broad front; we do everything we can. We ignore the people who promise an instant and easy fix—drugs don't work.

Tackling one of the risk factors of metabolic syndrome is tough—taking on all of them might seem overwhelming. But aggressive lifestyle changes and, in some cases, medication can improve all of the metabolic syndrome components. The goal of treatment is to reduce the risk of heart disease and diabetes. A doctor will recommend lifestyle changes or medicines to help reduce your blood pressure, LDL cholesterol, and blood sugar. Getting more physical activity, losing weight and quitting smoking help reduce blood pressure and improve cholesterol and blood sugar levels.

CHAPTER 2

WHAT CAUSES
DIABETES?

When we try to pick anything out by itself,
we find it hitched to everything else
in the universe.
—JOHN MUIR

D r. Roger J. Williams, the brilliant professor and discoverer of the B-vitamin pantothenic acid, introduced what is known as the genetotrophic concept: some problems of nutrition are hereditary. On the other hand, the World Health Organization says that healthy diet, regular physical activity, maintaining a normal body weight and avoiding tobacco use can prevent or delay the onset of type 2 diabetes at least. So what causes diabetes: genes or lifestyle?

GENETICS

Diabetes does not follow simple patterns of inheritance. However, it is clear that some individuals are born with a greater chance of developing diabetes than others. Even though type 1 diabetes and type 2 diabetes are different, there are two common factors affecting both: an inherited disposition to the disease and many environmental factors that contribute to the development of the disease.

Type 1 Diabetes

In the majority of type 1 diabetes cases, individuals have inherited a high-risk gene variation from both parents. Genetic variations are common, of course, and are not necessarily harmful —for example, different blood types are the result of gene variations. However, because many different genes influence an individual's risk of developing diabetes, the inheritance patterns of the disease are complex. There are many research projects that are currently being conducted to find a method of understanding and predicting an individual's predisposition to developing type 1 diabetes. Still, due to the complexity of the gene-gene and gene-environment interactions, it is difficult to accurately determine a person's true risk of developing the disease.

Most individuals with type 1 diabetes have been found to have variation in the human leukocyte antigen (HLA) complex of genes. This region contains several genes that make proteins responsible for helping the immune system to distinguish between the body's own cells and foreign invaders, such as bacteria or viruses. When this fails, there is an autoimmune reaction in which immune cells mistakenly attack healthy body cells, such as those of the pancreas.

One gene variation in particular in the HLA complex has been linked to diabetes. This is the DR form of the gene. HLA-DR is involved in several autoimmune diseases, disease susceptibility, and disease resistance. To make matters more complicated, however, different variations of DR affect people differently according to their ancestry. Caucasians are believed to have a greater risk of developing type 1 diabetes if they have gene variations known as HLA-DR3 and HLA-DR4, while people of African descent are thought to be at risk by carrying HLA-DR7, and those of Japanese heritage appear to have an increased risk with HLA-DR9. Even the difference between HLA-DR3 and HLA-DR4 can influence factors such as whether an individual develops diabetes earlier or later in life. This is extremely complex, but it is going to be a very important part of future real health care: personal, predictive, and preventive.

A person's risk of passing on the type 1 diabetes gene variations to his or her children depends on gender: men with type 1 diabetes have a 1 in 17 chance of passing on the high-risk gene variations; women who are younger than 25 years old when they give birth to a child has a 1 in 25 risk of passing on the high-risk genes, while women who give birth after the age of 25 have a 1 in 100 chance. This risk is doubled if one parent developed the disease before they themselves were 11 years old and increases to 25 percent if both parents have type 1 diabetes.

Approximately one in every seven individuals with type 1 diabetes also has a condition called type 2 polyglandular autoimmune syndrome (PGA II). A combination of type 1 diabetes and PGA II can cause thyroid disease, poor adrenal gland function, and other autoimmune disorders. If parents have these conditions, the likelihood of passing on the condition(s) to their children is 1 in 2. In my opinion, and with enough anecdotal evidence, this autoimmune syndrome is like most others—it would not occur if we avoided environmental and lifestyle factors that can affect gene expression, including diets high in sugar and refined carbohydrates, dairy products, and alcohol; massive inappropriate vaccination schedules; excessive antibiotic use; and both environmental and pharmaceutical chemical exposures.

Type 2 Diabetes

As with type 1 diabetes, many genes can affect the inherited risk for developing type 2 diabetes, and it is difficult to identify exact gene variations that can cause the disease. A number of polymorphisms in genes controlling metabolism are associated with an increased risk of type 2 diabetes. Determining a person's predisposition for type 2 diabetes is further complicated because the condition is actually caused by a complex interplay of genetics and the environment resulting in insulin abnormalities, increased glucose production in the liver, increased fat metabolism, and hormonal imbalances in the intestine.

The discovery that variation in the transcription factor 7-like 2 (TCF7L2) gene increases susceptibility to type 2 diabetes has been an important step in understanding this form of the disease. In fact, TCF7L2 has emerged as the most significant gene in the development of type 2 diabetes. TCF7L2 is found in pancreatic islets, which contain insulin-producing beta cells, as well as adipose (fat) tissue. Variations in TCF7L2 are associated with impaired glucose secretion and increased glucose production by the liver, as well as an increased risk of conversion from pre-diabetes to diabetes and a greater chance of gestational diabetes.

Another gene called KCNJ11 has also been linked to diabetes. It appears that variants of this gene impair the insulin response to glucose, so that inadequate levels of insulin are produced or secreted and blood glucose levels remain high. In adults, gene variation increases the risk of type 2 diabetes. A variant of KCNJ11 is also known to be responsible for about one third of the cases of permanent neonatal diabetes (NDM), a rare form of the disease that develops within the first six months of life.

Because type 2 diabetes is, to some extent, inherited, individuals whose mother or father has type 2 diabetes have a risk of developing diabetes themselves. Also, at the time of diagnosis, over 50 percent of people are obese and the rest are usually overweight. Again, the trends to obesity and overweight are partially inherited but the genes that are responsible are strongly influenced by diet and exercise. At this stage there are many other genes that come into play and the problem becomes extremely complex. However, there are many things one can do to reverse this downhill spiral.

The new sciences of epigenetics and nutrigenomics offer great hope to people who have type 2 diabetics. This means that diet and lifestyle changes specifically tailored to the individual's gene polymorphisms can influence gene expression, possibly reversing the disease process. Clinical advances in these fields are being made at a very rapid pace, and without the need to wait for long periods for drugs to be developed. The best treatments can be achieved with vitamins and other nutrients that improve the way genes are expressed.

MATURITY ONSET DIABETES OF THE YOUNG

It's worth mentioning another, though less common, type of diabetes that is hereditary. Maturity Onset Diabetes of the Young (MODY) is a form of the disease that typically occurs first during adolescence or early adulthood, although it sometimes remains undiagnosed until later in life. Whereas type 2 diabetes is caused by variations in several genes at once, MODY is caused by a variation in a single gene. However, there is more than one type of MODY, and the kind that an individual develops depends on which gene is affected.

In MODY, the pancreas can produce insulin, but insulin secretion from the pancreas is impaired. People with MODY may have only mild symptoms of diabetes and may not require insulin injections if they are able to control their blood glucose levels through diet and oral diabetes medications. They generally are not overweight and do not usually have other risk factors for types 2 diabetes, such as high blood pressure.

FOOD ALLERGIES

When I started studying medicine in the late 1960s, the only allergies that I was taught about were hay fever, possibly eczema, and very rarely asthma. By the time I started practicing medicine in the early 1970s, the idea that many symptoms people suffered were caused by food allergies and chemical sensitivities was still entirely disregarded by the medical profession. I became interested in the influence of food and chemical adverse reactions in a wide variety of patients, including those with arthritis, depression, schizophrenia, skin diseases such as psoriasis and eczema, chronic fatigue, and autoimmune diseases, including lupus and scleroderma. Still, by the 1980s, the concept that food allergies could cause or aggravate diabetes went largely unrecognized by the medical profession.

Still, over the last thirty years or so, there has been a slow but increasing recognition that allergies can cause other health problems. The recognized incidence of food allergies has increased from less than 1 percent to almost 20 percent. According to some of the best research available, food allergies are a clear risk factor for the development of type 1 diabetes. As discussed earlier, type 1 diabetes is believed to be caused by an autoimmune disorder in which the immune system mistakenly targets the body's own healthy tissues. There is evidence that certain proteins from some foods—including cow's milk and wheat and other grains that contain a protein called gluten—may stimulate immune cells called T-cells, causing them to attack the pancreas. In people with food allergies who also have gene variations that make them predisposed to type 1 diabetes, a low oral tolerance to particular foods will increase their chances of getting the disease if they consume these foods. In the future, testing for a low tolerance to specific foods could be an important means of predicting an individual's predisposition to diabetes.

When we examine food allergies, sensitivities, intolerances, and autoimmunity, we see many different types of reactions to allergens and irritants. There is what we consider a "true" allergic reaction from peanuts, which can cause severe anaphylaxis and death; abdominal discomfort from milk due to lactose intolerance; and the development of a cancer called lymphoma in patients who have celiac disease. These various reactions depend on genetics and environment and include the presence of known allergies, hormone levels, level of physical activity, physical and mental stress, viral infections, long-term parasitic infections, and—most important from the nutritional and orthomolecular medicine point of view—deficiencies of vitamins, minerals, trace elements, fatty acids, and other important micronutrients.

I group all of the Adverse Reactions to Ingested Food and Chemicals together under the umbrella term ARTIFAC. It is very difficult to identify the all of the foods and chemicals that may trigger allergies, sensitivities, intolerances, and/or autoimmunity in specific individuals. Any symptom in the medical textbook, from head to toe, may be caused by ARTIFAC. There are various tests available to measure antibodies that are produced by the immune system in reaction to certain foods and chemicals. These tests are called RAST (radioallergosorbent) and ELISA (enzyme-linked immunosorbent assay) tests, but they are very limited in their ability to make an accurate diagnosis.

Celiac disease is an autoimmune disorder that is caused by a protein called gluten found in wheat and gliadin, a breakdown product of gluten. There is an increased risk of diabetes in patients with celiac disease. Researchers have discovered antibodies to wheat gluten and gliadin in people with type 1 diabetes, meaning that these people have an abnormal immune response to wheat proteins. However, it is not necessary to have full-blown celiac disease to be sensitive to gluten and possibly other wheat proteins. It is highly likely that the processing food undergoes is creating serious health hazards by changing the nature of the ingredients in foods and increasing their potential for allergy. This is another very powerful reason for consuming fresh, whole, unprocessed foods. I have a patient who needs only to eat a crumb of bread and she bleeds bright red blood from the bowel. She has celiac disease and mild colitis—at least for the time being.

It is becoming increasingly apparent that an allergy to cow's milk puts individuals at an increased risk of developing diabetes. Nearly 100 percent of newly diagnosed type 1 diabetics have antibodies in their blood to the proteins in cow's milk. Japanese researchers have discovered that people with type 1 diabetes have very high levels of antibodies called IgA to certain proteins.

The allergies that have been studied the most by the Japanese are cow's milk proteins called bovine serum albumin and beta-lactoglobulin. From my understanding, the proteins and peptides in cow's milk can have a strong sedative effect on the nervous system and powerful psychological effects, as well. I believe that some individuals can become highly addicted to these foreign proteins, and may even suffer from psychiatric illness as a result. I have frequently used the term "milk madness" in my clinical lectures. But when it comes to diabetes, the problem is not the nervous system but the immune system suffering the bad reactions to cow's milk.

We now know that the early introduction of cow's milk feeding to infants increases the risk of children developing type 1 diabetes, and researchers have developed an understanding of why this may be so. Cow's milk and cow's milk formulas contain small amounts of bovine insulin. When a baby is fed cow's milk containing bovine insulin, it will produce antibodies to the cow's insulin, called anti-insulin antibodies. It is possible and highly probable that these anti-bovine insulin antibodies could attack the insulin-producing cells of the pancreas, or the infant's own insulin. This is the basis of autoimmune disease, which is believed to be the main process causing type 1 diabetes.

Exclusive breastfeeding for at least six months can provide protection against type 1 diabetes in childhood, as well as against childhood cancers such as leukemia and lymphoma, and childhood allergies. My recommendations are for mothers to breastfeed for at least six months and preferably twelve months—the longer the better. Both of my children were breastfed until three years of age. I have insulin dependent diabetes in my family history. My children were not introduced to cow's milk until after 12 months of age and even then it was limited. As adults, they both dislike cow's milk.

Based on experience and science, I believe the foods that have the most damaging effects on children with type 1 diabetes are sugar; cow's milk and its products; yeast; wheat and white flour products; and other grains that contain gluten, such as barley, rye, and oats. Citrus fruits may also cause problems for children with diabetes who have evidence of upper respiratory allergy such as hay fever, a sticky fluid build-up in the middle ear called glue ear, and/or a constantly runny nose. If we eliminate these foods from the diets of children who have diabetes, we would see healthier children.

I have treated many patients who were suffering symptoms of allergies and autoimmune disorders. Without a doubt, they benefited when we removed allergens—typically foods or food additives and chemicals—from their diet and environment. This required admitting the patients to the hospital and putting them on a four-day fast, which meant they ate nothing for four days and drank water only. During that time they were closely observed and at the end of the fast they would be given one food at a time—a food "challenge"—three times a day. Observations of the patients made before during and after the food challenges included the appearance of any symptoms, pulse rate, blood pressure, grip strength, fine motor movement, and blood glucose levels. These tests were done every fifteen minutes for two hours following the food challenge.

While observing one of the schizophrenic patients who had just finished a meal of bread only, I noticed that his blood sugar levels remained exceedingly high for a very long period of time after eating. I suspected that he had an unusual reaction to the bread, because after two and a half hours his blood sugar level plummeted to way below normal and his mental state deteriorated so severely that he required high-dose injections of a sedative to settle him down. I concluded that some foods in some people elevated blood sugar levels for prolonged periods.

It wasn't long after this experience that I admitted some of my diabetic patients into the same hospital, closely observing them during a four-day fast, and then introducing the food challenges. Initially the patients were type 2 diabetics; later I introduced the same testing program to mild type 1 diabetics who required only low doses of injectable insulin. Interestingly, the same patterns of high blood sugar occurred after some of these food challenges—and it was not necessarily high-sugar foods that caused high blood sugar levels. For example, one patient had a massive increase of blood sugar level from a normal 5 millimoles per liter to a very high 18 mmol/L after consuming a meal of zucchini, which is actually quite low in sugar. I can only conclude that this patient had a unique reaction to this particular food. Another had extremely high blood sugar levels after eating stone fruits (for example, cherries, plums, apricots, nectarines, and peaches) but not other fruits. When we eliminated the stone fruits and a few additional foods, she was fine. Many patients with whom I worked reacted extremely badly to dairy products. Wheat and other cereal grains and breads caused abnormally high blood glucose in other patients. The reasons for this are not fully understood, but there is definitely an individual and genetic component to it.

I believe that we should not take any allergy or ARTIFAC lightly in anyone, especially a diabetic. The study looked at several cases, including a 66-year-old woman with type 2 diabetes who had a history of multiple drug and food allergies and developed a severe allergy of the lungs, asthma and giant hives when started on human insulin therapy, and then developed chest pain and electrocardiogram (ECG) changes; a 55-year-old woman who had no history of cardiac disease who exhibited severe skin allergy after eating shellfish and then developed chest pain and shortness of breath upon cessation of the allergy; a 49-year-old healthy male who developed chest tightness and mild shortness of the breath (dyspnea) 24 hours following an allergic skin reaction to an antibiotic; a healthy 50-year-old man who sought medical attention for an anaphylactic reaction to multiple bee stings and developed chest pressure in the emergency room which showed a heart attack. Coronary angiography, the use of a dye and x-rays to view the arteries to the heart, was performed on these patients, and others showing significant narrowing (greater than 70 percent) in one or more of the coronary arteries. These

FOOD ALLERGIES AND DIABETES: A CASE HISTORY

Gay was a 42-year-old clerk who enjoyed life to the fullest including an overeating and over drinking program that she was proud of. She was 5 foot seven in height and weighed 82 kg. She had been referred by her general practitioner to a specialist in diabetes because of an elevated blood sugar level. The fasting blood glucose level was 13 mmol per liter and she was told that she may need to go on to insulin injections. When she came to see me she was in a desperate state. She had been placed on a complex carbohydrate diet and oral medications to bring her blood sugar down and this was the cause of her anxiety. Her fasting blood sugar levels had reduced to between 9 and 10 mmol per liter but the specialist was unhappy with the progress. Gay was willing to be admitted to hospital to undergo a fast, no food and only water to drink, followed by food provocation testing. The reason that we decided to go along with the food allergy pathway was that Gay had suffered from irritable bowel syndrome and knew that certain foods upset her. Some foods made her extremely tired. The only relevant past history was that she had gallstones and mild eczema as a child. Gay underwent a series of large bowel enemas to remove any food residues, followed by a series of food challenge tests to see if any foods caused clinical signs or symptoms. The food challenge tests involved eating a single food three or four times a day. Each time the food chosen would be different starting with low allergy foods such as rice, pears and lamb. As each food was introduced the nursing staff would record whether or not Gay suffered from any symptoms such as tiredness, brain fag, irritable bowel, nausea, headache, skin itch etc. Every fifteen minutes her pulse rate, blood pressure, blood sugar and grip strength would be measured. The insulin levels were also monitored on the hour.

It was determined from the above tests that Gay was sensitive to cows milk, stone fruits and the vegetable zucchini. In fact it was these fruits and cows milk which commonly caused her symptoms. However one of the most fascinating of the test results was the fact that the zucchini, which is not high in sugar or carbohydrates, caused her blood sugar to soar from 6 mmol per liter to nearly 16 mmol per liter. This was a very unexpected outcome. We repeated the test for the zucchini and the result was the same. This reinforces the whole notion that individuality is a crucial factor in nutrition. Exactly what the mechanism is by which the zucchini causes such a massive rise in blood sugar is unknown. It may be that the zucchini influences the pancreas and reduces its insulin output, or it influences the liver and stimulates it to produce more sugar, or it may be that the zucchini contains a natural chemical substance that blocks the effect of the insulin.

A salient lesson from these observations is that no two diabetics are nutritionally the same or even immunologically the same. This reflects the wide genetic variation in human illness and disease and that one size does not fit all; diabetics may respond to drug or insulin treatment but that does not mean they are cured or have optimum health.

Gay adopted an elimination diet and was given the nutrients that she was deficient in. She lost over 20 pounds in weight over the next three months and was able to stop the drugs for her diabetes. Interestingly, her pancreas showed signs of recovery in that her insulin levels returned to normal in hospital following the removal of the foods that she was sensitive to. We know that cows milk can have a serious adverse effect on the human gut. It is the most common cause of chronic stubborn constipation in infants. The pancreas is just an outpost of the gut and there are good reasons to believe that cow's milk may shut down the pancreas.

There are lessons in this case history that should be taught to every medical student and doctor in the world. And there are lessons from this case, which should direct best quality research into the future; the lessons being that allergenic foods can cause diabetes and insulin production/activity can be improved by removing offending foods and supplying the correct nutrients.

patients underwent successful revascularization surgery and recovered without complications. It is thought that in these ARTIFAC individuals, the allergic reactions produce the chemicals of allergy (ARTIFAC) that magnify the problem of the blocked arteries.

ENVIRONMENT/LIFESTYLE

Genetics alone is not enough to cause diabetes, and having a high genetic risk does not guarantee that an individual will develop the condition. The strongest evidence for this is displayed in cases of identical twins, where one develops diabetes and the other does not. Identical twins have identical genes but, interestingly, research has shown that when one twin develops type 1 diabetes, the other twin develops diabetes only about 50 percent of the time. In the case of type 2 diabetes in identical twins, when one twin develops diabetes, the other twin has a 75 percent chance of developing the condition. Thus, while genetic inheritance can increase the risk of diabetes, an individual's environment and lifestyle also contribute in large part to the development of the disease.

There are several external factors that have been linked to the development of type 1 diabetes in the presence of high-risk genes. For instance, cold weather is theorized to have an effect, because diabetes tends to develop more often in winter than in summer. Also, as mentioned above, food allergies can increase the risk of developing diabetes in people who are already predisposed to the condition. Excessive psychological stress or physical stress—injury or illness, exposure to chemicals, or a binge on drugs and/ or alcohol—can overwhelm the immune system and trigger a response that may cause the white blood cells to attack and destroy the beta cells in the pancreas that produce insulin. However, by far the biggest contributing factors to the development of diabetes—in particular, type 2 diabetes—in recent times are interrelated: poor diet (high in fat, sugar, and refined carbo-hydrates), sedentary lifestyle, and obesity.

Diet

People who eat lots of refined, processed foods—typically rich in fat and sugar, low in protein and fiber—run a higher risk of developing type 2 diabetes. Consuming large amounts of refined sugar, such as juices rich in fructose and soft drinks high in sucrose (common sugar), places stress on the pancreas, liver, and other organs, and can predispose an individual to diabetes. Multiple nutrient deficiencies—not uncommon, of course, in people who eat a lot of nutrient-poor foods—are also believed to contribute to the development of diabetes. These include low levels of vitamins C and E; the minerals magnesium, zinc, and chromium; and omega-3 fatty acids (fish oils), to mention only a few. This risk of diabetes is increased for people who also lead a sedentary lifestyle (see below). By contrast, high-risk individuals who eat a healthy diet and exercise regularly can reduce their risk of developing the condition.

Sedentary Lifestyle

People who lead a sedentary lifestyle are more prone to diabetes, when compared with individuals who exercise. Even moderate exercise a few days a week can make a real difference.

Obesity

Obesity is one of the strongest risk factors for type 2 diabetes, and it is often—although not always—linked to a nutritionally poor diet in combination with a sedentary lifestyle. Like diabetes itself, obesity appears to have some genetic basis, although it is strongly influenced by external factors, as well. Several key genes are currently used as markers for genetic predisposition.

The Beta3-adrenergic receptor gene, which is found in deep fat cells, makes a protein in that is involved in determining metabolism—in other words, how the body uses fuel for food. A defect in this gene, called TRP64ARG, reduces the activity of the Beta3-adrenergic receptor gene, slowing metabolism and the rate at which fat is burned. The result is a tendency toward obesity. The defective gene is not present in all people with type 2 diabetes, but it can influence development of the disease. It is also more common in Pima Indians and other populations with a very high incidence of type 2 diabetes.

Researchers have discovered that a variant in a gene called FTO can also affect metabolism and weight gain. The FTO gene makes an enzyme called fat mass and obesity-associated protein that is expressed in the hypothalamus (a control center in the brain), the pancreatic islets, the pituitary gland, the adrenal glands, and fat tissue. Although the exact function of the FTO gene has not yet been identified, studies have shown that people who have type 2 diabetes are more likely to have a particular variant of the FTO gene that is associated with obesity. And, as we know, obesity itself is a risk factor for diabetes. In particular, the gene variation of FTO is linked with elevated body mass index (BMI); waist circumference; fat mass; and leptin, a protein-hormone that reduces appetite. There is also a relationship between individuals who have two copies of the variant with physical inactivity and whole body insulin sensitivity.

Although the mechanism is different than that of FTO, genetic variation in insulin-induced gene 2 (INSIG2) has been implicated in obesity, as well. This gene makes a protein that inhibits the body's manufacture of fatty acids and cholesterol. It is believed that people who have a particular variation in INSIG2 are less able to curb the synthesis of fatty acids and cholesterol, and may therefore gain weight more easily than people who do not have the gene variation.

Inflammation is thought to play a role in development of both obesity and type 2 diabetes. Studies have shown that levels of an inflammatory protein called interleukin-6, regulated by the IL6 gene, are chronically elevated in people who are obese and/or who have type 2 diabetes. There are several gene variations in IL6, and there is evidence that these variations are connected to insulin resistance; high blood levels of fatty substances, such as cholesterol and triglycerides, also known as dyslipidemia; and metabolic syndrome, which we will discuss in Chapter 2. Numerous studies have also investigated the effects of exercise on the expression of IL6 gene variation. These studies have found that after six months of aerobic exercise, "good" HDL cholesterol increased and body fat, intra-abdominal adipose tissue, and fasting insulin decreased.

The peroxisome proliferator-activated receptor gamma gene (PPARG) regulates fat cell development, fatty acid metabolism, and insulin sensitivity—all of which are negatively affected in type 2 diabetes. Gene variants reduce PPARG function and can result in the development of insulin resistance, decreased diastolic blood pressure, and altered serum triglyceride levels, which may explain the correlation with type 2 diabetes. Interestingly, several studies have demonstrated the risk independent of an individual's body mass index. Furthermore, research has also demonstrated that individuals who presented with the two copies of the non-variant gene were actually protected against type 2 diabetes.

The fatty acid binding protein 2 (FABP2) gene makes a protein that is involved in fatty acid absorption and metabolism. A variation in this gene results in high levels of unhealthy fat molecules, such as triglycerides, that are a link between obesity and insulin resistance in some individuals with type 2 diabetes. It is yet to be determined what extent FABP2 gene variation has on obesity compared to external factors such as diet and exercise.

A variation in the lipoprotein lipase (LpL) gene is linked to coronary artery disease (CAD) and type 2 diabetes. A variation in the gene for the calpain-10 (CAPN10) protein have been shown to affect insulin secretion that may play a vital role in type 2 diabetes . However, as it is only a recent finding, there has been some disagreement regarding the significance of the data. So you can see that this is a very new science and there will be debate about the interpretation of scientific discoveries in genetics for a very long time.

HYPERTENSION

It had been reported in many studies that there is direct relation between hypertension and diabetes. The two conditions occur together so frequently that they are officially considered to be "co-morbidities"—diseases likely to be present in the same patient. In fact, diabetes and hypertension share a common set of risk factors, notably obesity, poor diet, and sedentary lifestyle. Unfortunately, high blood pressure makes diabetes even more dangerous and diabetes makes high blood pressure more difficult to treat. For example, diabetes can affect the elasticity of blood vessels, causing them to stiffen and, as a result, increasing blood pressure. If we apply logic and reason, it's clear that both diabetes and hypertension may be better controlled with diet, exercise, and nutritional supplementation. These natural prevention and treatment measures could decrease or eliminate the need for pharmaceuticals.

There is evidence pointing toward a genetic component to hypertension. A polymorphism in the gene encoding the G-protein beta 3-subunit (GNB3), which transmits information from receptors on cells to several proteins, increases systolic blood pressure (SBP). In addition to hypertension, this gene variation has been linked to cardiovascular disease, obesity, certain psychological syndromes, insulin resistance, some cancers, and a variety of immunological responses in various populations. Interestingly, an increase in geographical latitude—that is, moving farther away from the equator—reduces the amount of GNB3 gene variation. The is actually a worldwide variation in people's blood pressures. At low latitude, SBP is low and the frequency of the GNB3 is high. At high latitude (that is, nearer the poles), SBP is high and the frequency of GNB3 is low. To put this in perspective, this refers to individuals north of the 43rd parallel in the Northern Hemisphere (Marseille, France; Rochester, NY; Vladivostok) or south of the 43rd parallel in the Southern Hemisphere (Hobart, Tasmania; Christchurch, New Zealand), who have the GNB3 gene variation are at higher risks of developing hypertension. Individuals who have lower latitude of origin cannot attribute hypertension to this polymorphism. However, hypertension everywhere in everyone can be improved with diet, exercise, nutritional supplementation and stress reduction.

Other Factors

Age

Increased age is a factor that gives more possibility than in younger age. This disease may occur at any age, but 80 percent of cases occur after 50 year, incidences increase with the age factor.

Serum Lipids and Lipoproteins

High triglyceride and cholesterol levels in the blood are related to high blood sugar. High blood sugar increases risk even with low LDL levels in circulating blood.

Gestational Diabetes

Women who have had gestational diabetes run a greater risk of developing type 2 diabetes later in life. The genetics associated with gestational diabetes is often complex and is currently not well understood. However, women who have a family history of diabetes are more likely to develop gestational diabetes, particularly if the heredity is through their maternal line. As in other forms of diabetes, environmental factors contribute to the development of gestational diabetes, and the risk increases with age, weight, and overall well-being.

We cannot just blame diabetes on our genes, or on our geography. And, we cannot take a magic single pill, nutritional or pharmaceutical, and be done with it. Diabetes is complex, and intelligent management involves a total lifestyle approach. This can include appropriate medication along with the suggestions made in this book. Common sense caution: work with your physician, and do the tests and measures you need to get results. In addition, tell your doctor that you want a therapeutic trial of nutrition and other non-drug approaches to find out to what extent they help you. Have your doctor monitor your progress. You may find that your need for medication is reduced. In fact, it is likely. The big question is, by how much? Stay with me—we will be discussing this in the chapters to follow.

CHAPTER 3

DIABETES DIAGNOSIS AND TREATMENT

Learn and live. If you don't, you won't.
—U.S. ARMY TRAINING FILM,
WORLD WAR II

HOW IS DIABETES DIAGNOSED?

Diabetes was first "discovered" when ancient physicians diagnosed diseases by tasting a patient's urine for sweetness. Thankfully, doctors today have machines to do this. According the World Health Organization (WHO), if there are symptoms of diabetes such as excessive thirst and frequent urination combined with a raised blood glucose level after fasting overnight, or a high blood glucose level two hours after drinking a glucose solution, the person has diabetes.

There are several tests that are used to diagnose pre-diabetes and diabetes. Three of the most common tests are addressed here.

Fasting Plasma Glucose (FPG) Test

The fasting plasma glucose (FPG) test measures blood glucose in a person who has not eaten anything for at least eight hours. It is most reliable when done in the morning. People with a fasting glucose level of 7.00 mmole/L per liter of blood (mmole/L) or above are diagnosed as having diabetes.

Oral Glucose Tolerance Test (OGTT)

The oral glucose tolerance test (OGTT) also measures blood glucose after a fast of at least eight hours. However, in this test, blood glucose levels are measured immediately before and again two hours after the person drinks a beverage containing 75 grams of glucose. Diabetes is diagnosed if the blood glucose level above 11.1 mmole/L. Research has shown that the OGTT is more sensitive than the FPG test for diagnosing pre-diabetes, but it is less convenient to administer.

By the time a blood glucose test is performed there has generally been a long period during which the newly diagnosed diabetic has had a sugar problem. I believe that this sugar challenge test should be performed more regularly. It can be used to predict diabetes a long time before the diabetes develops. For example, if during the test the blood sugar level goes up very high and then suddenly drops down, there is a problem. The sudden drop in blood sugar occurs because the pancreas pumps out a large quantity of insulin to bring down the high level of blood sugar, and in the process the insulin supply is exhausted. This places tremendous stress on the pancreas. Over many years, the pancreas weakens and finally fails to produce enough insulin to meet the body's demands. This is diabetes.

Incidentally, after the surge in insulin and rapid drop in blood sugar, the patient frequently suffers from many symptoms associated with functional reactive hypoglycemia, or low blood sugar. Symptoms include nervousness, anxiety, weakness and fatigue, lightheadedness, confusion, sweating, palpitations, blurred vision, and headaches. Unfortunately, if hypoglycemia has been a problem for many months or years, diabetes may be just around the corner.

Glycosylated Hemoglobin Test

The glycosylated hemoglobin test, also known as the hemoglobin A1c (HbA1c) test, measures an average of blood sugar levels over a period of several months. Glycosylation is a process by which sugar that is not used for energy attaches itself to hemoglobin, a molecule in red blood cells that transports oxygen in the bloodstream. The more glucose there is in the bloodstream, the more glucose builds up in the cells. Because red blood cells typically live in the bloodstream for about four months, the HbA1c test measures the amount of sugar that has become attached to the hemoglobin in red blood cells over a period of time. Chronic, uncontrolled high blood sugar levels cause cell damage, poisoning cells so that they cannot function properly.

HbA1c results are given as a percentage. Normal levels of A1C are below 6 percent. Higher levels of A1C, from 6.5 percent and up, indicate poor blood glucose control.

WHAT TREATMENTS ARE AVAILABLE FOR DIABETES?

The goal of diabetes treatment for all forms of the disease is to keep blood glucose levels consistently within a healthy range, minimizing high blood sugar levels while keeping them from dipping too low. Type 1 diabetes is treated foremost with insulin, along with diet and exercise, whereas type 2 diabetes is treated first with weight loss, diet, and exercise, and medications—such as oral diabetes medications or insulin—only if the other measures are not effective.

It is claimed that neither type 1 nor type 2 diabetes can be cured. However, I will show in this book that most people who have type 2 diabetes can be cured and come off all or most medications if they chose to change their lifestyle—eating a healthy diet, beginning a program of regular exercise, and taking nutritional supplements. It is far more difficult to reverse type 1 diabetes to this extent, although some people have been able to stop their insulin while many, if not most, can reduce their need for insulin. The importance of eating a healthy diet that includes lots of whole, raw foods and few (if any) products containing sugar and white flour, as well as limiting alcohol, cannot be over-stated. Taking vitamin, mineral, and other nutritional supple-ments is also key in any diabetes treatment plan, as we will see in coming chapters.

Diet

People who have diabetes, like all of us, may suffer from a wide range of allergic symptoms that they often believe are untreat-able. These symptoms can include physical and mental fatigue; irritability and moodiness; recurrent headaches; generalized aches and pains; stomach pain and irritable bowel syndrome; cough-ing, sneezing, and congestion; itchy skin; and more. One of the most effective ways of determining if a food is causing a prob-lem is to try an elimination diet, such a lamb, rice, and pear diet. These are all foods that are generally regarded as safe and rarely cause adverse reactions. It is then a matter of introducing one food at a time each day and recording whether or not typical symptoms occur. Here we are looking for foods that affect the general health and well being of people with diabetes; we are not looking for the foods that cause the diabetes.

Improving general health will help to relieve the stress of many of the symptoms of diabetes, including high blood sugar. As men-tioned earlier, some of the most common foods thought to cause many of the symptoms in people with ARTIFAC are dairy prod-ucts, wheat and other cereal grains, yeast, and citrus fruits. Other sources of allergy symptoms include nuts (especially peanuts), chocolate, and shellfish. It is interesting to note that in most stud-ies on allergies, common old toxic sugar is never included, nor are beverages such as coffee, tea, and alcohol. Sometimes it's sim-ply a matter of removing sugar and chemical additives—color-ings, flavorings, and preservatives—from the diet and many of the uncomfortable symptoms of food allergies will disappear or at least become more tolerable.

As somebody once said, "Individuality is a crucial factor in nutrition." This is so true in diabetes. No two people with diabetes are the same; each should be given an individualized treatment plan based on his or her food reactions. In some instances, blood sugar levels could be brought under control by removing offending allergens through an elimination diet and instituting a dietary plan that included raw foods, whole foods, and limited refined and complex carbohydrates. However, most patients also had nutritional deficiencies and required supplementation with vitamin C, B-complex vitamins, minerals, and other nutrients in order to manage their diabetes. The majority of patients who enter a clinic, doctor's office or hospital will be suffering nutritional deficiencies, nutritional imbalances and ARTIFAC. Unfortunately for everyone, doctors rarely make these diagnoses.

A fascinating observation became noticeable during my work with diabetic patients: I discovered that if the patients remained on an elimination diet and supplementation program, the amount of insulin produced by the pancreas would increase and stay at reasonably normal levels. I observed these same results in patients who had required insulin before the diet and supplement treatment and who were able to stop the insulin injections or reduce the dose once the treatment had taken full effect. This means that adjusting diet and nutrient supplements according to individual needs gave the pancreas an opportunity to recover. Exactly how this can come about is not fully understood. We know that there are some vitamin supplements, as discussed elsewhere in this book, that can protect the pancreas from ongoing damage and may restore the insulin-producing cells. We also know that vitamin C and other supplements can improve the function of insulin produced by the pancreas. It is likely that allergens could be switching off the action of the pancreas and/or blocking the effects of the insulin it is producing. These areas of human health require a lot more research. Otherwise, we will be relegated to looking for more and more drugs to treat sicker populations.

Over the last decade, a vast of amount of money and energy has gone into researching the effects of the food components of traditional diets in combating the killer diseases of modern civilization, such as cardiovascular disease and diabetes, and its precursor metabolic syndrome. A strong emphasis of this research has been on the Mediterranean region. The Dietary Approaches to Stop Hypertension (DASH) diet and the Mediterranean Diet, like many healthy-eating plans, limit unhealthy fats and emphasize fruits, vegetables, fish and whole grains. Both of these dietary approaches have been found to offer important health benefits—in addition to weight loss—for people who have components of metabolic syndrome. Ask your doctor for guidance before starting a new eating plan. Components of the Mediterranean diet—grapes, berries, wine, olive oil, garlic, fish, nuts, and legumes—have all demonstrated spectacular healing benefits either alone or in combination. Many of these foods have been identified as containing compounds that exert anti-obesity, anti-diabetic, anti-inflammatory, and cardio-protective affects. Some notable examples are the anthocyanidins from berries, resveratrol from grapes, and sulfides and other bioactive compounds from garlic. In fact, the sulfur compounds found in garlic influence the HMG-CoA reductase enzyme, an action similar to that of statin drugs but without the harmful side effects. The most active compound in garlic is vinyldithiin and can be obtained in a stabilized form.

Recent research has also shown that the carotenoids from edible seaweeds, catechins from green tea, polyphenols and theobromine from chocolate, curcumin from turmeric and the components of cinnamon also display activity that can benefit people with metabolic syndrome. Many of these compounds are now available as dietary supplements, which in many instances offer greater bioavailability and efficacy.

Exercise

We all know that moderate exercise helps so many things, and

THE GLYCEMIC INDEX

Despite the controversy that this concept has caused, research has consistently shown that an effective dietary measure for reducing fat mass is to reduce the sugar load, also known as the glycemic load, in the diet. To quote University of Sydney Medical School professor Jenny Brand-Miller, "The past 2 years have seen a steady stream of reports indicating that restriction or modification of carbohydrate intakes can favorably affect weight loss and cardiovascular disease (CVD) risk factors." My take on this is: no sugar, white flour products, or alcohol, and a minimum of complex carbohydrates, which means no carbs after lunch if you want to lose weight. This does work.

Recent clinical trials have shown that both high-protein and low-glycemic index diets increase visceral fat loss. Probably the easiest way to decrease sugar load is to maintain a relatively high ratio of protein to carbohydrate at each meal, with carbohydrates coming almost entirely from vegetable sources. This ratio is all-important. There should be an emphasis on good protein sources, such as lean meat and fish, to increase satisfaction, decrease appetite, and reduce cravings for high-sugar foods such as bread, biscuits, pastries, potatoes, and so forth. Not only does this increase insulin sensitivity and improve the use of the energy from foods, but it also influences the brain's appetite circuit, effectively switching off the appetite centers in the brain—no more hunger, just a normal appetite.

we all have so many excuses to "not exercise today." I tell my patients to do appropriate, regular exercise if they want to get well and stay well. It is your free choice whether you personally will exercise today or if you will not. Please make the life-saving decision.

Sleep

Research conducted into this area is beginning to show that sleep duration may be an important regulator of body weight and metabolism. Links have been found between the daily (circadian) rhythms and key components of energy balance, body heat production, hunger or satiety and the sleep-wake cycle. Sleep debt has a harmful impact on sugar metabolism and hormone function.

Levels of hormones that control the appetite and your energy balance are leptin and ghrelin. They are altered when you are deprived of sleep. Participants in a study who slept for five hours had 15 percent lower leptin levels and 15 percent higher ghrelin levels than those who slept for eight hours. The brain interprets a drop in leptin as a sign of starvation; so it responds not only by boosting hunger, but also by burning fewer calories. That means you put on more weight even if you don't eat any more food.

In another study is was shown that when twelve healthy young men were restricted to just four hours of sleep for two consecutive nights, their leptin levels were 18 percent lower and their ghrelin levels were 28 percent higher than after two nights of sleeping for ten hours. One of the principle authors of this study, Professor Eve Van Cauter, Ph.D., was quoted as saying that this level of sleep deprivation brought the participants close to a pre-diabetic state. Quite profound, quite correct.

A comprehensive, inclusive and integrative management strategy to combat Metabolic Syndrome is inevitable in a health system that has to all intents and purposes ignored the counsel of the wise and produced a generation of children who will, if they don't die before their parents, become a colossal disease burden unto themselves.

Friendly Bacteria and Immunity

The lining of the small intestine is called the mucosa. The mucosa secretes digestive enzymes and mucus that protects the mucosa from invading bacteria and viruses. The mucosa also has white blood cells and immune cells to attack invading bacteria and neutralize the harmful effects of foreign proteins that may escape into the bloodstream. Alterations to the immune system in the mucosa are associated with type 1 diabetes. This is likely to be a major contributor to the failure to form tolerance to foreign proteins. As a result, autoimmunity is established; that is, the immune system breaks down and attacks its host, the diabetic.

In 2008, a publication from the American Diabetes Association included a story titled "The Perfect Storm for Type 1 Diabetes," which supported the practice of nutritional and orthomolecular medicine. This involves the replacement of harmful bacteria in the stomach and intestines through a more vegetarian diet and probiotics; the repair of very small holes in the gut wall with nutrients such as vitamin C, zinc, glutamine, and the herb golden seal; and the stimulation of the gut immune system and gut defenses with diet and nutrients, thus enabling the gut to function properly. This form of treatment may be applied to both type 1 and type 2 diabetes. The objective is to reduce the food allergy load on the immune system and reduce the likelihood of immune reactions to food having a bad effect on the pancreas and liver. The other objective is to make sure that the bacteria inside the gut are friendly and don't produce proteins and chemicals that the body reacts to; directly or indirectly aggravating the diabetes. It is well known that some bad bacteria in the gut can cause the immune system to produce antibodies. These antibodies attack the normal tissues of the body including connective tissue, the thyroid gland, the adrenal glands, the pancreas and even the meninges of the brain (the coverings of the brain).

Another important issue with regard to the health of the intestines is toxins and poisons. We are constantly consuming toxins and poisons in our food and water supply. Drugs, medicines, alcohol, aspirin and even the breakdown products of sugar in excess can cause damage to the fine lining of the intestines (the mucosa). Therefore it is important to consider in the diabetic all of these aggravating factors and remove as many as possible.

Vitamins and Minerals

In nutritional medicine, often more than one nutrient will be required to correct a problem, especially with diabetes. The problem is that most doctors want a single silver bullet (a drug) to fix a problem. This is the reason that single-nutrient studies are potentially dangerous, because if a single nutrient doesn't fix the problem, one might conclude that it is of no use in that particular disease. As you will come to appreciate, diabetes is a disease in which many levels of many nutrients are low or even deficient. Thus, the use of only one or two vitamins or minerals may not achieve very much at all.

One of the most profound recent discoveries has been that vitamin D, administered at a dose of 2,000 international units (IU) per day, can reduce the risk of type 1 diabetes in children. We now know that this vitamin acts on cell nuclei, which con-

---

METRICS MADE EASY

International Units (IU) are a measure of biological activity. Grams, milligrams, and micrograms are measures of weight.

One gram (g) is 1,000 milligrams (mg). A gram of a powder is about a quarter-teaspoon.

A milligram is 1,000 micrograms (mcg).

And to keep this fun:

For those interested in the ancient history of Greece and Troy, a millihelen is the amount of beauty it takes to launch a single ship.

tain genetic material. Vitamin D may eventually be scientifically proven to have a positive effect even on high-risk genes. Also, children who are more prone to developing diabetes and who have an abnormally low insulin production after a sugar challenge, in addition to having antibodies to their beta cells, can be protected against developing diabetes later in childhood with megadoses of vitamin B_3 (niacin). There is still some controversy over this, however. The medical community does not fully understand that some individuals have the genes to respond to the vitamin B_3 by itself, while others will require other nutrients in addition to the B_3, such as vitamin E complex and/or fish oils. Controversies in medical science develop as a consequence of ignorance and inexperience in the science of nutritional and orthomolecular medicine.

Nutritional supplements are recommended for all diabetics. There is not a single diabetic who will not benefit from appropriate and judicial supplementation. It is medical negligence to ignore the scientific literature on the health benefits of supplementation in prediabetes, types 1 and 2 diabetes, gestational diabetes, metabolic syndrome and those with a genetic predisposition to diabetes.

We will consider other nutrients and herbal remedies later on in this book.

PART 2

NUTRITIONAL SOLUTIONS

Supplements confer huge benefits to the present and long-term health of people suffering from diabetes and all the other conditions mentioned above. Attempts to correct these deficiencies and imbalances with diet alone is at best unscientific and at worst gross medical negligence. It is about time that doctors were properly trained in Nutritional Medicine before they are ever unleashed onto the public.

To correct imbalances and deficiencies that contribute to suboptimal diabetic and metabolic control and to prevent diabetic complications should be the aim of every physician. This does not mean that orthodox medicine should be ignored, but in diabetes, it should be relegated to second place in every instance except for the severe diabetic and those with an urgent need for intensive hospital care, e.g., diabetic ketoacidosis, coma, etc.

These doses are the doses commonly used by Nutritional and Orthomolecular Medicine specialists and should not be used or self-prescribed by patients. These doses must be prescribed and monitored by qualified experts.

Individuals who may wish to use these supplements should do so with due care including the observation and adherence to the doses recommended on the label and the avoidance of supplements causing drug interactions if the person is taking the relevant drug.

In brief, these supplements perform the following functions:

- protect the pancreas and other organs from the damaging effects of free radicals

- increase the likelihood of the pancreas to make, store and release more insulin

- enhance the activity of the insulin available to the body's cells

- provide high levels of antioxidants to slow the aging process and retard progression of diseases and their complications

- support and stimulate the immune system to fight infection and reduce the damage caused by any autoimmune process

- reduce the risks of cancer, heart disease, stroke, kidney disease, eye disease, osteoporosis, gangrene and killer infections

- reduce cholesterol and triglycerides

- improve wound healing

- increases mental and physical well-being enabling effective exercise to be performed

- provides important anti-inflammatory and pro-healing nutrients to allow the resolution of chronic inflammation in the deep fat of the gut

CHAPTER 4

VITAMIN C:
THE MIRACLE WORKER

Discovery consists of seeing things that everyone else sees,
but thinking what nobody else has thought.
—ALBERT SZENT-GYORGYI, M.D., PH.D.

We all know the story about a disease called scurvy that killed thousands of sailors at sea, and how this disease was cured with a simple citrus fruit. The fruit contained a substance called the anti-scorbutic factor, which was later isolated and given the name ascorbic acid. Today ascorbic acid is more commonly known as vitamin C.

Vitamin C is not a true vitamin—it is actually a six-carbon molecule that has the ability to perform miracles in mankind. Almost all living things can produce vitamin C, or ascorbate, intrinsically in the body from glucose. Those that cannot produce ascorbate include humans, the higher apes, guinea pigs, Indian fruit bats, and a species of salmon; thus, these creatures must obtain vitamin C from the diet. But because stress—including the stress of an illness such as diabetes—depletes levels of vitamin C, the diet simply cannot provide enough ascorbate to satisfy the body's needs. As a consequence, we have another vicious cycle in which the diabetes creates an increased need for ascorbate but the diet is not adequate in its provision of the nutrient. Therefore the diabetes gets worse, the ascorbate becomes more depleted, and the diabetes continues to deteriorate.

From its own self-evident worth, ascorbate has become one of the most popular nutritional supplements in the world. Despite this, and the fact that there are over 60,000 scientific papers and medical studies pointing to the benefits of ascorbate, it is still not regarded by medical doctors as a serious treatment for ill patients. In fact, it should be used routinely, in sickness and in health. However, the medical establishment in general is trained to think and act in terms of disease—to make an orthodox diagnosis and prescribe drugs or surgery to cure. Diet and nutrients are ignored and, as a result, the true health and fitness of the patient is ignored.

There is a pandemic of nutritional imbalances and deficiencies worldwide, especially in the Western industrialized countries. These imbalances and deficiencies are particularly evident in patients with metabolic syndrome, pre-diabetes, and diabetes. It doesn't take an Einstein to diagnose nutritional deficiencies in an overweight or obese patient who has poor skin conditioning, dark circles under the eyes, and dull hair, and who complains about fatigue and a lack of energy. Yet, when this same person goes to the doctor, what is the solution? Medical tests, a diagnosis and drugs. This is not good healthcare—this is simply medical care. And while it may be world's best medical practice, it is actually contributing to the massive increase in diabetes and other degenerative diseases worldwide.

It is a pity for all of us that the medical profession has control of our health systems. The emerging paradigms of integrative medicine and nutritional medicine will change this dangerous situation. In the meantime, the first thing anyone who has prediabetes or diabetes should do is to begin supplementing with at least 1,000 milligrams to 4,000 mg of ascorbate per day. For people with diabetes, dietary sources of vitamin C simply aren't enough to meet the body's needs. One of the issues is the inability of body cells to respond to the insulin that is available. This makes low levels of vitamin C even more problematic, because insulin actually helps to transport vitamin C from the blood and body fluids into the cells. The conclusion here is that all of the cells of a diabetic are deficient in vitamin C, and so—because vitamin C is the most important antioxidant—the cells, tissues, and organs are chronically degenerating due to oxidative damage.

The classic vitamin C deficiency disease is scurvy, in which a long period of tiredness, fatigue, and muscle aches occurs before the more characteristic symptoms appear, including easy bruising and bleeding gums. The period of time from an absolute ascorbate deficiency until the more serious signs of scurvy is about two months. Most of us obtain sufficient vitamin C from the diet to prevent the full-blown serious end-stage disease of scurvy. This is true even for diabetics. However, many of us suffer from a mild form of scurvy, or subclinical scurvy, with generalized symptoms such as tiredness, fatigue, and muscle aches and pains. This simply means that our cells and tissues are not receiving adequate amounts of ascorbate to allow them to function optimally. It is also one of the main reasons why diabetics tend to develop so many complications, such as frequent infections, heart disease, atherosclerosis, kidney disease, and eye disease.

Over the millennia, there have been literally thousands of epidemics of scurvy, which have occurred mainly in the winters when fresh fruits and vegetables are not readily available. It is also likely that, during these times of scurvy (or "pre-scurvy") epidemics, immune function was weakened in entire populations, creating an ideal environment for the development of plagues or pandemics of killer infections. While we don't see these more obvious scurvy epidemics occurring in wealthy nations, another epidemic is affecting us. This is the epidemic of subclinical scurvy, in which the majority of the population is simply not taking in enough vitamin C. It is one of the major reasons we see so many instances of degenerative disease—and diabetes is just the tip of the iceberg. It took more than sixty years after James Lind discovered ascorbate's use in preventing scurvy at sea for the British

Admiralty to order that lime juice be given to its naval crews. Today, neither the medical profession nor the general public appears to have fully recognized the importance of ascorbate in the functions of day-to-day living. Yet this miraculous substance is preventing disease in hundreds of thousands of people and saving countless lives through the practice of nutritional and orthomolecular medicine.

Vitamin C should be given to every patient, whether his or her symptoms are physical, psychological, psychiatric, or traumatic. Of course, all of these classes of symptoms may apply to a person who has diabetes. An assessment of a diabetic's overall health must include a measurement of vitamin C levels in the system before determining a treatment plan. The best test is the measure of vitamin C in white blood cells, which will reveal accurately whether or not a patient has subclinical scurvy or low levels of ascorbate contributing to the diabetes. It is interesting to see the improvement in well-being and the reduction of symptoms, both psychological and physical, in diabetic patients who are given a few vitamins and a large dose of vitamin C. It is also fascinating to learn from these patients that their diabetes specialist has reduced the amount of insulin they need to take because their blood sugars have fallen. Unfortunately, the specialist usually shows very little interest in the vitamins and nutritional treatments.

HEALTH BENEFITS OF VITAMIN C

Most diabetics have a mild form of vitamin C deficiency called subclinical scurvy, and will require supplementation with vitamin C to achieve optimal health. The diabetic's health care provider (preferably a nutritional and orthomolecular medicine specialist) will determine the optimal daily dose. If the diabetes is severe enough and there are complications, the physician may discuss with the patient the possibility of using intravenous vitamin C to address the problem initially. Intravenous treatment will saturate the body with vitamin C more quickly than taking oral doses. For example, if the patient is suffering from recurrent infections, poor wound healing, hypertension and heart failure, severe anxiety and depression, and signs of poor circulation in the feet and toes, it is imperative that treatment with intravenous vitamin C is undertaken immediately.

Excess glucose in the blood is toxic. It poisons body cells, fats, proteins, enzymes, and genes, changing their structure and reducing their functionality. This sugar poisoning is responsible for causing most of the damage and complications in diabetics, including widespread damage to the heart and blood vessels supplying the brain, kidneys, and other vital organs. Vitamin C not only helps to block this activity, but also cleans up the damage caused by high glucose levels. In this way, ascorbate can reduce kidney, nerve, and eye diseases, and other diabetes complications. The use of vitamin C has saved or prolonged the lives of many diabetics all over the world through its broad spectrum of activity. It has also improved quality of life by preventing the development of diabetic eye disease and cataracts.

To my mind, it is irresponsible and bordering on malpractice when a physician neglects to test for vitamin C deficiency and fails to prescribe vitamin C for diabetic patients. Using vitamin C in the treatment of diabetes not only makes sense scientifically, but also economically. Only 1 to 2 grams (1 gram is 1,000 mg) of vitamin C per day is enough to rid body cells of a toxic substance called sorbitol, which poisons the nerves and delicate tissues of the eye.

Heart Disease

Vitamin C is one of the most powerful and widespread active antioxidants in the body. Among its many other actions, this incredible nutrient reduces "bad" LDL cholesterol, increases "good" HDL cholesterol, strengthens the connective tissues of the heart and blood vessels, lowers blood pressure, and prevents platelets in the blood from adhering too much to each other. Vitamin C even improves the activity of other antioxidants, such as beta-carotene and vitamin E.

Atherosclerosis is a primary cause of cardiovascular disease, which is a general term for conditions including heart attack and stroke. It begins with damage to the delicate tissues that line the arteries, such as by oxidized LDL cholesterol being deposited in the arterial walls. White blood cells attempt to digest the fatty cholesterol deposits in order to "clean up" the site; however, what results is a plaque—an accumulation of cholesterol, immune cells, and debris that can harden over time, narrowing the arteries and reducing blood flow to the heart. Even more dangerous, pieces of the plaque can break off and travel through the blood stream to smaller blood vessels, where they may become lodged and cut off blood flow to tissues and organs. This is a common cause of heart attack and stroke. Atherosclerosis affects not only the heart and brain, but also the lungs, intestines, kidneys, and extremities.

When it comes to treating atherosclerosis in a person with diabetes, it is never too late to begin treatment with vitamin C. A word of caution here is important: If there are deficiencies of nutrients such as magnesium, zinc, copper, chromium, and B-complex vitamins, then the activity of vitamin C in more severe cases of atherosclerosis is limited. This does not mean that vitamin C should not be given; instead, it means that the other deficiencies must be corrected, as well. This also applies to people with diabetes who have high blood pressure. Vitamin C supplementation is, of course, essential, but a possible magnesium deficiency must be addressed, as well. Generally, the higher the dose of vitamin C, the more blood pressure is reduced (to a certain point). Patients on medications for hypertension should continue taking the drugs at the same time as beginning supplementation with vitamin C. Closely monitoring a patient's blood pressure will allow the physician to slowly reduce the dosage of blood pressure medication. The patient may even be able to stop it after three to six months.

Two other nutrients that are helpful in treating heart disease and diabetes are vitamin D and calcium. Calcium plays a role in reducing blood pressure and vitamin D is important for the absorption of calcium from the gut. People with diabetes who need to take insulin are at greater risk of arterial damage, because insulin actually contributes to the hardening of the arteries. If the arteries to the heart are severely affected, a heart attack may result. If the blood vessels that supply the brain are affected, a stroke may occur. If damage is to the kidneys, the patient may need dialysis. If it is to the legs and feet, gangrene may develop, leading to a need to amputate toes, feet, and even the entire leg in order to save the patient's life. Therefore, any patient with diabetes who show signs of poor circulation in the toes and feet (or anywhere, for that matter) should be given enough vitamin C to relieve those symptoms. If there is no relief of symptoms, the use of the chelating agent EDTA and magnesium will assist in opening up the circulation to the affected toes, foot, or leg.

Immunity

Diabetics tend to get more infections than non-diabetics, and these infections are frequently more severe and difficult to treat. Vitamin C plays a critical role in immune system function by supporting white blood cells that kill invading viruses, bacteria, and fungal infections. Without adequate levels of vitamin C, these white blood cells cannot function adequately. When there is an infection, the white blood cells consume huge quantities of vitamin C while they are destroying the invaders. If the amount of vitamin C in the white cells falls below a certain level, these immune cells fail and the infection grows worse. And vitamin C is not the only nutrient that is consumed—the other antioxidants in the body become stressed, as well, and they are also destroyed by the infection. If this process continues, the patient will develop a more severe infection, such as pneumonia, or die.

Very high doses of vitamin C have been used in extremely

severe viral and bacterial infections with the result that patients at risk of dying have been saved. Usually these doses are so high that they must be given intravenously in order to reach the high levels necessary to kill invading germs and stimulate the white blood cells. Furthermore, patients with diabetes, cancers, leukemias, and many other degenerative diseases are at high risk of infections to begin with, because the diseases themselves reduce the levels of vitamin C in the body cells.

The important message here is that no matter how sick a diabetic patient may appear, high doses of intravenous vitamin C will give that patient a far better chance of beating the infection and staying alive. I have used megadoses of vitamin C in the treatment of thousands of patients, including many diabetics suffering severe life-threatening infections, and I have seen the vitamin save lives after drugs and antibiotics have failed. Sadly, the opportunity to receive this limb- and life-saving therapy has too often been denied to too many diabetics.

Should a doctor or hospital refuse to allow the patient access to nutritional therapies, my advice to the patient (or to the family if the patient cannot act on his or her own behalf) is to seek legal action immediately, and to direct that action toward the hospital and its management. One cannot in these circumstances afford to entertain a debate about the pros and cons of intravenous vitamin C with doctors who are inexperienced in its use. Patient lawyer to hospital lawyer is the recommended path. There has been more science published to support the use of high doses of vitamin C in the treatment of a wide range of conditions than any other substance or drug. There is no drug that works like vitamin C, which has a proven ability to: improve white blood cell activity; increase immune chemicals in the blood; stimulate antibodies and immune hormones; strengthen resistance to invading germs; selectively kill cancer, melanoma, and leukemia cells without harming normal cells; increase glutathione in the brain; and relieve depression and some schizophrenias. There is no drug on the planet for which a dose can safely be increased by over 1,000 times its normal dose. By contrast, vitamin C can be given in megadoses, which helps it mount a powerful immune response to beat infections.

While there remains a great deal of controversy over the benefits of vitamin C, science and scientists do not generate this controversy. It is generated by a medical profession that is heavily dependent on drugs and the pharmaceutical industry for its existence. There are other health professionals outside of the medical profession who are more interested in assisting the body to heal itself. It is these health professionals whose advice should be sought when it comes to the use of nutritional supplements and, in particular, the use of intravenous vitamin C. Some alternative, complementary, and integrative health professionals, including some doctors, may also have misgivings about the use of intravenous vitamin C. In these circumstances, the diabetic patient should refer to some of the references and organizations at the end of this book for better advice and help.

There are many other nutrients that work with vitamin C in strengthening the immune system and fighting infections. A raw food diet high in vegetables, plus good quality protein such as fish and eggs, will provide many of the nutrients that will help vitamin C to boost immunity. However other supplements are often necessary, for added benefit, including zinc, selenium, copper, carotenoids (from carrots, pumpkin, and other yellow and orange vegetables), flavonoids, vitamin E, and some amino acids. An amino acid complex called glutathione works very well with vitamin C in diabetics, but it is best given by intravenous injection for severe cases. There are forms of glutathione that can be taken orally and that are not broken down by the acids in the stomach. However these are quite expensive supplements and should be reserved for the times when they are needed. There are also quite a number of herbal medicines (discussed later in this book) that can help improve immunity.

Infertility

In the Western world, there is an increasing incidence of infertility in both males and females. People who are overweight or obese and who have diabetes or are at high risk of developing the disease are more likely to be infertile. High blood glucose levels, which cause sugar poisoning, are partly responsible for this, because excess sugar can inactivate male sperm and cause harm to the female egg. However, losing weight and taking a reasonably high dose of vitamin C can reduce toxic sugar levels and improve fertility in couples. Vitamin C actually protects the very highly active sperm from oxidative damage to the DNA. In order to become pregnant, it is critical for people of childbearing age who have diabetes—and especially those with type 1 diabetes—to bring their blood sugar levels under strict control while at the same time supplementing with vitamin C. Other nutrients are also important in supporting fertility, of course, especially in men. These include a balance of essential fatty acids (fish oils), zinc, selenium, and vitamin E complex.

VITAMIN C SAFETY

Most forms of vitamin C are extremely safe if taken in the recommended doses. Depending on the country in which you live, the recommended daily allowance ranges from 50 mg to 100 mg, so you may be surprised to learn that 220,000 mg has been given intravenously over a period of twenty-four hours period *without any adverse effects*. This was the dose that I gave HIV patients to defeat infections and the Kaposi's skin cancers. This enormous dosage is the exception to the rule. Most patients, even very sick ones, respond to less. But "less" is still a lot more than you might think.

A patient with swine flu on life-support had completely shut down kidneys and lungs: yes, neither the lungs nor kidneys were working. He was given 100,000 mg per day of intravenous vitamin C. This is over 1,000 times the recommended daily dose. His lungs cleared, his kidney function returned to normal and his leukemia disappeared following the treatment with the massive dose of intravenous ascorbate. The leukemia had not returned at the time of writing this book, over eighteen months later. In my experience, it will not return provided he stays on a high oral dose of vitamin C and is given injections in the case of illness or trauma. The reason that I mention this case is that it was the subject of two *60 Minutes* television shows in New Zealand in 2010 illustrating how powerful intravenous vitamin C is even when all else has failed. The shows also illustrate how the mainstream medical profession can offer only flimsy excuses when they are challenged with a life-saving vitamin therapy. These shows can be viewed on the Internet; I have provided the links in the Bibliography.

During medical school I was taught that doses over 100 mg per day would cause kidney stones and/or kidney damage. This teaching still continues today in many medical schools, and it is the reason that most doctors graduate completely ignorant of the miraculous healing power of vitamin C. The best proof of the vitamin's safety, however, is that over the last thirty years, many hundreds of thousands of high-dose vitamin C intravenous injections have been given to a large number of patients in the United States, Canada, South America, Europe, and Australia, without kidney damage or stones forming. In fact, in many Asian countries—especially India, Vietnam, and parts of China—intravenous vitamin C is given routinely to treat infectious diseases.

The myth that high doses of vitamin C would cause kidney stones and kidney damage has come about because, theoretically, ascorbic acid can be converted to a substance called oxalic acid, which combines with calcium in damaged kidneys to produce kidney stones. Vitamin C itself does not cause kidney stones. Kidney stones form in damaged kidneys, if there is too much calcium in the urine, too much uric acid (gout patients), and a number of medical drugs. If your doctor wants to test your urine for oxalic acid crystals, then ensure that he or she acidifies the urine and freezes it before it goes to the lab. Otherwise, the test result will show that there is oxalic acid in the urine when there should not be.

Another myth surrounding vitamin C is that it can destroy vitamin B_{12} in the body. While it does interfere in the laboratory with the test for vitamin B_{12}, the fact is that people who take vitamin C often have higher levels of vitamin B_{12} in their blood. It would seem that a medical doctor who was against the use of vitamin C supplements created this myth. His work was condemned and he lost his credibility.

Some medical professionals have claimed that when vitamin C is withdrawn from treatment, a form of scurvy called "rebound scurvy" occurs. My colleagues and I have never witnessed this in clinical practice. Furthermore, when a person such as a diabetic has a real need to be taking oral doses of vitamin C—for example, to prevent or treat complications—then it is for that very reason that long-term low, moderate, or even high doses of maintenance vitamin C should be continued. If it works, why withdraw it?

Some cancer specialists have frightened patients away from the use of high-dose oral vitamin C and intravenous vitamin C because they claim that it interferes with chemotherapy and radiotherapy. This is nonsense. Many studies and much experience with use of high doses of vitamin C in seriously ill patients (including diabetics and diabetics with cancer) confirm its extreme usefulness. In Australia, when this fear failed to work with many patients who had strong beliefs in the benefits of vitamin C, the oncologists would insist that patients not take vitamin C injections because they claimed it destroyed the veins used for the chemotherapy. One thing is for sure—vitamin C has virtually no damaging effects on the veins if used properly, whereas chemotherapy is extremely destructive. The message I am trying to convey here is that the medical profession will attempt to rationalize its position regarding the use of vitamin C with reasons and logic that are baseless and make very little scientific sense.

There are only a few reasons why high doses of vitamin C should not be given for fear of kidney damage: if the patient has had recurrent kidney stones in the past, if the patient has severe kidney disease and is on haemodialysis, or if there is a history of severe gout with the formation of uric acid kidney stones. If the patient has severe kidney disease and is not on haemodialysis, then small doses of oral vitamin C may be used and, in fact, slowly increasing the dose may actually improve kidney function. Here we are talking about giving the patient between 100 mg and 1,000 mg per day initially. Should kidney function improve on these doses and with continued close monitoring of kidney function by a physician, then higher doses may be attempted—again, under close supervision—until a level of oral vitamin C is reached where no further renal function improvement can be achieved. There are many doctors, like myself, around the world who have seen the benefits of vitamin C and how it can improve the function of the organs that are typically affected by diabetes.

Types and Dosages of Vitamin C

Vitamin C supplements come in many forms, as powders, tablets, capsules, liquids, and gels. There are different chemical forms of vitamin C, including ascorbic acid, sodium ascorbate, calcium ascorbate, magnesium ascorbate, and potassium ascorbate. Most forms of vitamin C are absorbed by the body in a very similar way. I recommend a mixture of all of these different forms most of the time, but for high doses, it is safest to use a combination of ascorbic acid and sodium ascorbate. The only safe form that can be given intravenously is sodium ascorbate, because ascorbic acid is too acidic and destructive to the body's tissues, and the calcium, magnesium, and potassium salts of vitamin C can interfere with nerve transmission and heart rate, and—if given at high doses intravenously—may cause cardiac arrest.

You may wonder about the amount of sodium contained in sodium ascorbate, and its use in patients with diabetes and high blood pressure or kidney disease. However, the sodium in sodium ascorbate is handled different by the body and kidneys than the sodium in sodium chloride (table salt). Sodium in vitamin C is easily excreted by the kidneys; furthermore, the ascorbate component of vitamin C actually acts as a mild diuretic that helps to push sodium out of the kidneys and into the urine. Please do not forget that fast foods and junk foods, which contain large quantities of sodium chloride, are directly responsible for many cases of diabetes. The fact is that 15 grams of sodium ascorbate contains about 1.3 g of sodium. The average American or Australian consumes approximately 4 g of sodium per day as sodium chloride—this is equivalent to 10.1 g of table salt per day. So you can see that a reasonably high dose of 15 g of sodium ascorbate does contribute some sodium, but not at a level that is of concern for a diabetic patient who elects to make dietary changes, including not adding salt to food.

Some new forms of vitamin C combine the water-soluble vitamin with a lipid (fatty substance) that aids in the transport of the vitamin C from the intestine and into the bloodstream. It is claimed that these forms of vitamin C are almost as good as the injections. And for most diabetics who do not have complications or severe infections, these forms may be good enough. However, if the condition is serious enough, then this form will not be sufficient and injections will be the only effective treatment. I have created a table at the end of this book that gives the dosage schedules of vitamin C for diabetics and the particular complications of the disease that may occur. The range of vitamin C is between 2,000 mg per day and 100,000 mg per day, depending on the age severity, condition, and complications that the diabetic may suffer.

It is important to note that when the dose is increased to above 4 g per day, there is a trend toward a reduced absorption of the vitamin C by the gut. That is, the more vitamin C you take, the harder it is for the gut to absorb. However, there is still significant absorption even when doses at 10 to 20 g per day are taken by mouth. Vitamin C should be administered intravenously if there is a need to raise the body's tissue levels very high.

I am a physician, but I am not your physician. It is important that you work with your doctor on this. Your first task may be to get him or her to even give the idea a nod. Be informed, and be prepared for disagreement. It is your body. Vitamin C is too useful to dismiss out of hand.

CHAPTER 5

THE B-COMPLEX
VITAMINS

When in doubt, try nutrition first.
—ROGER WILLIAMS, PH.D.

One of the problems with our modern diet is that important vitamins, minerals, and trace elements are processed right out of our food. The removal of wheat germ and fiber from the wheat grain results in high-calorie white flour that lacks essential micronutrients. This becomes a real problem when white flour and white rice are staples in the diet. Over a long period of time, eating a diet that contains nutrient-poor processed foods can cause relative vitamin and mineral deficiencies and deficiency diseases. These are the degenerative diseases of industrialized societies—diseases of malnutrition that, ironically, result from overconsumption, made possible by the food industry and profitable for the pharmaceutical industry.

VITAMIN B₁ (THIAMINE)

Vitamin B₁, also called thiamine, was the first B vitamin to have been discovered. A deficiency of thiamine causes a disease called beriberi, which results in severe fatigue, muscle wasting, difficulty walking, mental confusion, fluid retention, high blood pressure, and heart failure. Although the severe form of beriberi is very

75

uncommon these days, milder forms of the disease are quite prevalent, and may cause some of the symptoms above, most notably high blood pressure, and mild to moderate heart failure—both of which are also common in diabetes. Patients are often treated for heart failure with drugs, when a high dose of thiamine and some of the other B complex vitamins plus heart nutrients such as coenzyme Q_{10} would correct the underlying problem. Other symptoms of low thiamine levels include depression, mild fatigue, sensations of pins and needles and numbness in the legs, and constipation. Generally, these deficiency symptoms are due simply to low intakes of the vitamin B_1. The symptoms of these milder deficiencies in diabetics respond extremely well to moderately high doses of vitamin thiamine. One of the most effective ways of treating constipation in the elderly, for example, is to give them a B complex vitamin that includes at least 100 mg of vitamin B_1.

Vitamin B_1 is essential for the body's production of energy from the carbohydrates in foods. It is particularly important in helping to provide energy for the nervous system. Low levels of thiamine in diabetics can result in poor mental functioning, difficulty with thinking and making calculations, and difficulties with communication and social relationships. A severe deficiency of vitamin B_1 may result in mental disorders. Unfortunately, deficiencies of vitamin B_1 and other B complex vitamins are more often than not overlooked in patients with diabetes. People with diabetes who regularly drink alcohol are doing themselves a real disservice when it comes to their health, because alcohol actually destroys vitamin B_1 and many of the other B complex vitamins. A serious drinker who has diabetes and a deficiency of vitamin B_1 may end up with a very severe brain disorder called Wernicke's Syndrome.

Dosage

Thiamine is an extremely safe water-soluble vitamin that can produce remarkable effects, especially in relieving fatigue in diabetic patients and people who typically consume high quantities of alcohol, sugar, and other refined carbohydrates in the diet. The recommended dosage for the treatment of a thiamine deficiency in people with diabetes ranges from 100 to 500 mg per day; however, if there are severe complications with heart disease, heart failure, and neurological symptoms, the dose may need to be as high as 8 g per day. High doses above 500 mg per day should be given under the care and guidance of a nutritional or orthomolecular doctor.

VITAMIN B₂ (RIBOFLAVIN)

Deficiencies of vitamin B_2, or riboflavin, are not uncommon, and symptoms can be easily seen and felt. For example, an inflamed, red, and sometimes painful tongue that may be mistaken for an infection is actually more likely due to a vitamin B complex deficiency, made worse by a lack of riboflavin. Other symptoms include cracked lips, particularly at the corners of the mouth; anemia; sensitivity to light; poor vision; skin problems, such as greasy dermatitis and oily skin at the sides of the nose; and an itching or burning sensation in the lips, eyes, mouth, and nose. Riboflavin deficiency may also cause disorders in the lining of the lungs, bowels, and bladder. However, it is important to note that low levels of riboflavin may not produce any noticeable symptoms at all.

While vitamin B_2 is very important in diabetics, its supplementation is also useful because it stimulates another very important nutrient called glutathione, which is believed to protect the lens of the eye against the development of cataracts. Cataract opacities in the lens of the eye result in reduced vision and eventually blindness. The removal of cataracts is one of the most common surgical operations and one of the most costly to the health system. Cataracts can be prevented with the use of riboflavin and other nutrients; supplementation is an inexpensive and safe means of preventing cataracts in everyone, but especially in people with diabetes. It is known that riboflavin, the green-yellow pigment that colors the urine when you consume B complex vitamins, can also sensitize your skin to sunlight, so there is speculation that it may sensitize the tissues in the lens of the eye to light as well. So if you are going to take riboflavin, it should be taken in low doses in a multivitamin, along with high doses of both vitamin C and vitamin E to protect the lens of the eye from light and oxidation damage.

Dosage

The maximum recommended dose of riboflavin is between 5 mg and 10 mg per day.

VITAMIN B$_3$ (NIACIN AND NICOTINAMIDE)

Vitamin B$_3$ is also known as niacin (sometimes called nicotinic acid) and nicotinamide. Both of these forms are important for patients with diabetes for a number of reasons.

Niacin (Nicotinic Acid)

Niacin is useful in people who have diabetes because it improves the secretion of insulin from the pancreas and improves the sensitivity of insulin in the muscle and liver cells of the body. In a diabetic patient who is at risk of heart disease and stroke, high doses of nicotinic acid provide a very safe and effective treatment by reducing "bad" LDL cholesterol, increasing "good" HDL cholesterol, and reducing triglycerides and lipoprotein A. It is better than the statin drugs. Many major clinical trials have been conducted with nicotinic acid and it has been proven to reduce heart attacks by 27 percent and strokes by 26 percent. The other great benefit of nicotinic acid is that over a period of twelve months it can reduce the thickness of hardened arteries and dissolve the cholesterol plaques that build up on the inside of the arteries by slowing down the flow of blood to vital organs.

Dosage

The dose of the slow release form of niacin is 1.5 g at night. Higher doses of nicotinic acid, such as 3,000 mg per day, can improve cholesterol and triglyceride levels in patients with diabetes even if they have severe arterial disease, including arterial disease in the legs. If the very high dose of 3,000 mg per day is not well tolerated, the dose can be reduced; in this case, there will still be beneficial effects, but they may take longer to occur.

The acidic form of vitamin B_3 causes flushing and tingling sensations in the skin. I have taken a high dose of nicotinic acid and my face turned as red as a ripe tomato. The flushing can be extremely unpleasant and the sensations may be very uncomfortable. These side effects can be prevented by taking a slow-release form of the nutrient in combination with several grams of some vitamin C.

There is one caution that needs to be mentioned with nicotinic acid: it has been reported to sometimes cause raised blood glucose and may aggravate diabetes. In my experience, whenever a good nutrient causes a problem like this it is generally a reflection of some other deficiency or imbalance. These must be looked for and corrected. It may simply be a lack of vitamin C, zinc, chromium, or vitamin B_6. Careful monitoring by your physician should prevent raised sugars from nicotinic acid.

Nicotinamide (Niacinamide)

Nicotinamide is extremely useful in preventing the development of diabetes in pre-diabetic individuals, as well as in protecting against ongoing damage to the pancreas in those who have the disease. The nutrient was first scientifically proven to prevent diabetes in animals in the 1950s. Diabetes can result from an auto-immune reaction in which a person's own white blood cells attack healthy body cells and tissues, including the insulin producing cells in the pancreas. Nicotinamide appears to block this effect, protecting the pancreas from ongoing damage by white blood cells. It also acts as an antioxidant that protects islet cells from damage caused by oxidation and some of the toxic chemicals produced by the patient's own white blood cells.

For patients with type 2 diabetes who are not overweight but who have failed to respond to the usual oral diabetes medications, nicotinamide has been shown to improve metabolism and insulin secretion. This means that even if drug treatment fails, lifestyle changes, diet, and appropriate supplementation including the use of nicotinamide, can offer a powerful and natural treatment. Furthermore, supplements may actually improve the action of oral diabetes medications.

While nicotinamide may not work in every prediabetic and diabetic patient who requires insulin, every patient deserves a trial of nicotinamide. It is true that nicotinamide may work better for some patients, but this may be simply because their overall nutritional status is better. In other words, *all* patients should be eating a healthy diet and taking supplements to ensure that they are getting optimal levels of nutrients, which will ultimately offer the best opportunity of producing a positive outcome. For example, a patient who is given nicotinamide and only has a partial response will do better if his or her intake of the minerals chromium, zinc, and magnesium, along with vitamins E, C, and B complex, are all at optimal levels. Nutritional and orthomolecular medicine doctors understand the importance of all of these nutrients and do not regard the treatment of a diabetic with a single "magic bullet" as being best practice.

There is very good scientific evidence to show that nicotinamide restores the insulin producing cells of the pancreas. To do this, of course, there must be some insulin producing cells remaining after the damage that caused diabetes in the first place.

The fact that nicotinamide can actually improve the regeneration of the insulin producing cells of the pancreas is remarkable enough, but the idea that these regenerated cells can then produce insulin is one of nature's miracles. There are many patients who are taking high doses of nicotinamide and other micronutrients who would have been injecting insulin had they not sought alternative help. In fact, I have treated patients who have been taking insulin for a number of years and who have been able to reduce or cease their insulin as a consequence of the regeneration of the pancreas by optimal nutrition. Unfortunately, for many diabetics who have taken high doses of insulin for a long time, this is not possible. I believe that stem cell therapy will be the answer to this illness for these patients.

Dosage

A newly diagnosed insulin-dependent diabetic should begin treatment with a high dose of nicotinamide immediately, under the guidance and supervision of a healthcare professional. By itself, up to 3,000 mg per day of nicotinamide may help to extend a patient's freedom from the need to use insulin for a significant period of time. Indeed, in combination with a nutrient-rich diet and the antidiabetic supplementation program, taking nicotinamide may delay the need for insulin indefinitely. It is in such circumstances that both their diabetic specialist and a specialist in nutritional and orthomolecular medicine should carefully manage and monitor the patient.

Individuals who are susceptible to diabetes, especially early onset type 1 diabetes, may be treated with nicotinamide to actually prevent the development of the disease. Doses of between 1,000 mg per day and 3,000 mg per day are recommended. People who are susceptible to diabetes often show antibodies in their blood to the insulin-making islet cells in their pancreas. People who have a family history of diabetes and who also have a high sugar consumption combined with overweight or obesity should be tested for diabetes. (Refer back to Chapter 3 for more information on tests to detect prediabetes and diabetes.) This approach is especially important for children who may show a tendency to diabetes. If a child who is at high risk of diabetes can be prevented from developing the disease through dietary changes and nutritional supplements (in particular, a high dose of nicotinamide), the family and society in general can only benefit. This approach is simple, scientific, reasonably easy to implement, and very economical in the long run. Somebody once said, "Self-discipline is far less hampering than chronic ill health." This is especially so in the case of diabetes prevention.

With the advent of genetic testing over the last several decades, the ability to detect slight variations in genes called polymorphisms, which may respond to particular nutrient therapies, is becoming more of a reality. One day it will be a matter of routine, rather than a rarity, to test for genes and polymorphisms, and to determine if specific nutrients may benefit people with diabetes. Nutritional and orthomolecular doctors will be able to identify which patients will respond best to which nutrients and dietary changes simply on the basis of a swab of cells taken from the inside of the patient's cheek. Nicotinamide and nicotinic acid are two vitamins that definitely fall in the category of nutri-genomic substances—nutrients that affect the way genes work.

VITAMIN B$_6$ (PYRIDOXINE)

Vitamin B$_6$ (pyridoxine) has been used in treating fluid retention, premenstrual syndrome, and depression for many years, but it has many uses reaching far beyond those three conditions. It is another extremely important vitamin for the prevention and treatment of diabetes and its associated complications. Vitamin B$_6$ is essential for the production of blood cells, proteins, insulin, and other hormones and chemicals that are involved the proper function of the immune system. It is also necessary in transmitting information from nerve cell to nerve cell in the brain and nervous system.

People with diabetes (both type 1 and type 2) often have low blood levels of vitamin B_6, so it's important for all diabetics to supplement with this vitamin. Children who have diabetes, in particular, are susceptible to vitamin B_6 deficiency, and this can be very harmful in the long term. A deficiency of vitamin B_6 causes many problems including anemia, poor nervous system functioning, red tongue, cracked lips, and oily skin and eczema. A more severe deficiency of vitamin B_6 can cause epilepsy, depression, and high blood sugar (in other words, diabetes). Other conditions associated with low vitamin B_6 levels are carpal tunnel syndrome, morning sickness during pregnancy, asthma, premenstrual syndrome, and recurrent kidney stones. The flavor enhancer monosodium glutamate (MSG)—commonly added to Chinese food, soups, and processed meats—can cause symptoms that are worsened by vitamin B_6 deficiency. People who are sensitive to MSG may experience nausea, anxiety, severe thirst, heart palpitations, and a tingling sensation of the face and arms.

In people with diabetes, vitamin B_6 deficiency is related to a condition called diabetic neuropathy, in which nerves are damaged as a result of chronically elevated blood glucose levels. Over time, high blood sugar poisons body cells, interfering with the ability of the nerves to transmit signals and weakening the walls of small blood vessels that supply the nerves with oxygen and nutrients. Symptoms of diabetic neuropathy include numbness and/or a sensation of pins and needles in the feet, muscle cramps, and weakness. It is interesting to note that symptoms of vitamin B_6 deficiency and those of diabetic neuropathy are almost identical. In fact, vitamin B_6 actually helps to block the toxic process that causes neuropathy. It is often used in combination with other nutrients to help with this debilitating complication of diabetes, and can dramatically reduce the symptoms. Therefore, vitamin B_6 should be considered as part of the treatment for all diabetics.

Vitamin B_6 is a critical nutrient for brain function. It is needed for the brain cells to produce important chemicals called neurotransmitters, which carry signals that communicate information from one brain cell to another. One of these important neurotransmitters is called serotonin, but there are many other chemicals in the brain that depend on vitamin B_6 for their production. Vitamin B_6 levels are generally lower in people who suffer from depression. A deficiency of vitamin B_6 can result in severe depression, which most often does not respond very well to the use of antidepressant drugs. Antidepressants work by increasing serotonin levels, but these drugs don't affect other important neurotransmitters. Because vitamin B_6 is involved in the production of a number of neurotransmitters, its action is superior to medications that affect only one neurotransmitter. In a diabetic person who also has depression, supplementation with vitamin B_6 and other co-nutrients will help increase interest and activity in work, social relations, and life in general, and improve their diabetes management as a result. No drugs can achieve this level of scientific medicine and health care.

Osteoporosis is a common complication of long-term diabetes. The use of vitamin B_6 in diabetes can be beneficial in preventing osteoporosis, along with other nutrients that aid in protecting the bones against this condition.

Dosage

Good sources of vitamin B_6 include whole grains, bananas, yeast, sunflower seeds, and peas and beans. Vitamin B_6 is made more active by the minerals zinc and magnesium.

The recommended dosage for vitamin B_6 is between 50 mg and 300 mg per day. However, if necessary, the dosage can be taken higher than 300 mg per day. This must be done under medical supervision, preferably by a specialist in nutritional and ortho-molecular medicine.

The long-term use of high doses of vitamin B_6 by itself may actually cause a form of nerve toxicity; however, this toxic effect is reversible when the vitamin B_6 supplementation is discontinued. Taking vitamin B_6 together with a high-potency B-complex vitamin can also help prevent nerve toxicity. The dosage of vitamin B_6 that appears to have caused nerve damage has been between 500 mg and 3,000 mg per day. These are doses that have been taken for many months or years without being balanced by the other B group vitamins.

The mineral zinc is essential to ensure that supplemental vitamin B_6 is converted to its active form in the liver, so people who are taking vitamin B_6 must also take in adequate zinc, recommended at 15mg to 60 mg per day.

VITAMIN B_{12} (COBALAMIN)

Vitamin B_{12} is a water-soluble vitamin (as are the other B-vitamins and C) that is required for red blood cell formation, healthy nerve cell function, and DNA synthesis. In food sources, vitamin B_{12} is bound to proteins, and it is released when food is digested in the stomach. Once released, the vitamin combines with a substance called intrinsic factor, so that it can be absorbed into the bloodstream. The active form of vitamin B_{12} in human metabolism is called methylcobalamin.

Pernicious anemia is an autoimmune disease that causes a failure to produce intrinsic factor, resulting in an inability to absorb vitamin B_{12} properly. If pernicious anemia is left untreated, it causes vitamin B_{12} deficiency. This form of anemia is so severe that it results in the death from heart failure. Some diabetics develop pernicious anemia as a result of the immune system attacking not only the pancreas, but also the bone marrow. This is all part of the autoimmune break down, which occurs in many diabetics. If vitamin B_{12} is not administered by injection, these patients will die. While most diabetics do not develop pernicious anemia, the majority of them do develop an increased requirement for vitamin B_{12} over and above what they obtain in their diet. Without optimal levels of vitamin B_{12}, diabetic neuropathy may develop. As you now know, this also occurs with severe vitamin B_6 deficiency. So it is important, in patients who have feelings of pins and needles and numbness associated with nerve damage, that they be given injections of vitamin B_{12}.

Again, as with vitamin B_6, a low level of vitamin B_{12} is associated with mental depression. This is particularly common in older people who have diabetes. Just a few injections of vitamin B_{12} can significantly improve the mood of an individual with diabetes who also has depression, and may help prevent the need for antidepressants and their myriad side effects. Another important supplement for the treatment of depression and that may also help the diabetes, is a substance called SAMe, which will be discussed later.

Dosage

The methylcobalamin form of vitamin B_{12} is best for the treatment of brain and nerve diseases because this form of vitamin B_{12} easily penetrates into the brain and nervous system. It can have a very powerful effect, providing all the other nutrients that are required for proper brain and nerve function are at optimal levels. The dosages of methylcobalamin range from 1,000 micrograms (mcg) per day to 10,000 mcg per day. A microgram is 1,000th of a single milligram, so that dose could also be expressed as between 1 to 10 milligrams. Still, for most physicians, these are very high doses. High doses are sometimes necessary to achieve a good outcome. Vitamin B_{12} should never be given by itself; it must be accompanied by a reasonably high dose of folic acid, another B complex vitamin. In the most severe cases of diabetic nerve disease that do not respond to injections of methylcobalamin, the nutrient may be given as an injection into the cerebrospinal fluid (CSF), which, as the name suggests, is fluid that surrounds the brain and spinal cord. This procedure is undertaken only in special circumstances; it is not common.

Once the effect has been achieved with the use of intramuscular injections of methylcobalamin, it is wise to reduce the injections and give the patient a sublingual tablet that is placed under the tongue. Methylcobalamin B_{12} is absorbed reasonably well this way.

FOLIC ACID

Folic acid is probably best known for it for its role in preventing neural tube defects such as spina bifida in developing embryos, so supplementation is usually recommended during pregnancy. However, this nutrient has other important functions, as well. Although folic acid may not affect diabetes directly, it is very useful in preventing complications that are associated with diabetes, such as atherosclerosis, osteoporosis, and mental illness and depression. There are also some other conditions associated with diabetes in which folic acid may be helpful. For example, in celiac disease, the allergy to wheat protein can result in the body's inability to absorb vitamins and minerals from the intestine. As mentioned earlier in this book, celiac disease may lead to the development of diabetes. Therefore every patient who has diabetes and who has gastrointestinal symptoms should be tested for celiac disease and/or sensitivity to gluten, in addition to being screened for a wide range of vitamin and mineral and deficiencies.

Folic acid helps remove an amino acid called homocysteine that is toxic to virtually all tissues and organs. Homocysteine must be quickly converted to the safe amino acid, cysteine, to prevent tissue and organ damage. In people who have diabetes, it is extremely important to reduce homocysteine levels in order to lower the risk of cardiovascular complications, such as heart disease and atherosclerosis, which are more common in people with the diabetes. Folic acid requires vitamin B_{12} and vitamin B_6 to reduce homocysteine. In some people this is easy to achieve, while for others it may be quite difficult. It all depends on the individual.

Folic acid deficiency is very common. Deficiency can cause anemia, inflamed gums, poor growth in infants and children, an increased risk of infections, depression, loss of short-term memory, shortness of breath on exertion, fatigue, anxiety, and insomnia.

Dosage

Vegetables are the best source of folic acid, particularly dark green leafy vegetables such as spinach. It's important to note, however, that folic acid is easily destroyed by heat in cooking. Furthermore, there are many drugs, including alcohol, that interfere with action the action of folic acid, or even destroy the nutrient.

Folic acid is very safe, even at the high doses that are required to reduce the toxic amino acid homocysteine, and to elevate mood in depression. Folic acid and vitamin B_{12} should always be taken together. Taking one without the other can cause a serious imbalance and result in damage to the nervous system. Taken together they improve nervous system function.

In the case of folic acid deficiency, the first measure to address the problem is to increase the amount of green vegetables in the diet. This will not correct that deficiency entirely, but it will go a long way in helping. The advantage of including more green vegetables in the diet, particularly for people with diabetes, is that these foods are also a very rich source of magnesium, which is also more often than not required as a supplement, and fiber. The dose for people with diabetes can range from 500 micrograms (mcg) per day to 10,000 mcg per day. I routinely give 5,000 mcg of folate and 1,000 mcg to 5,000 mcg of vitamin B_{12} (by injection) to all diabetics I start them on a nutrition program. Combined with the other nutrients, the profound effects of B vitamins on the overall well-being of people with diabetes is almost a miracle—and with no adverse effects.

Dosages above 500 mcg per day of folic acid taken for more than a few weeks should be monitored by a qualified nutritional and orthomolecular doctor. When taken in doses above 2 mg per day, folic acid should be accompanied with regular injections of vitamin B_{12}. For the treatment of depression in diabetes, the dose may need to go as high as 5 to 10 mg per day. Extremely high doses of folic acid can cause a loss of appetite, nausea and increased flatulence, and may even aggravate depression, especially if vitamin B_{12} is not given with it. A suitable probiotic supplement (or yogurt) containing live friendly bacteria can be very effective in reducing these side effects and should be taken with two or three times per day with meals. Finally, the nutritional supplement called SAMe, which is important in helping depression, may also be of benefit to the diabetic by helping to improve liver function and detoxification.

BIOTIN

Biotin is a B vitamin involved in the production of energy. It is important in the manufacture and use of amino acids and fats, and it works with an enzyme called glucokinase in the liver to break down blood sugar. Glucokinase is either weakened or lower in concentration in diabetics, and biotin can improve the activity of the enzyme.

People who have diabetes tend to have lower than normal levels of biotin. Symptoms of deficiency include hair loss; brittle nails; dry, scaly skin around the eyes, nose, and mouth; nausea and loss of appetite; and greasy skin in some areas. Should a diabetic have any of these symptoms, a deficiency of biotin should be suspected and supplementation considered.

Dosage

Biotin is available from organ meats such as liver, kidney, and sweetbread (thymus or pancreas), as well as some cheeses. The "good" bacteria (probiotics) in the intestines can manufacture biotin from vegetables. Egg yolk and yeast are also rich sources of the nutrient. Keep in mind, however, that raw egg whites should never be consumed because they inactivate biotin.

The dose of biotin for a diabetic who develops symptoms such as scaly skin and brittle nails is between 500 mcg and 3,000 mcg per day. Because beneficial bacteria in the gut can manufacture biotin, it is important to maintain healthy levels of these bacteria through supplementation with *Bifidus* and *Lactobacillus,* as well as by eating a diet that is composed principally of fresh, raw foods. Doses of biotin may need to be higher for people whose diabetes is not well controlled. For people with type 1 diabetes, doses of biotin may need to be as high as 20 mg per day; people with type 2 diabetes will benefit from 10 mg to 20 mg per day.

While biotin is a very safe supplement, it should always be given with a high potency B complex vitamin, because the B-vitamins work best as a team. The use of other supplements such as carnitine and coenzyme Q_{10} will provide the building blocks for improved energy and health. However in the doses that are required to achieve this, the supplements become quite expensive. It is wise to take a small maintenance dose of biotin in the daily supplement routine.

CHAPTER 6

VITAMIN D

Go outside and play.
—EVERYBODY'S MOTHER

One of vitamin's D most important actions is to help the body maintain normal blood levels of calcium and phosphorus, two minerals that are essential for normal bone formation. As such, vitamin D has long been known to play an important role in building strong, healthy bones and teeth, and recommended daily intakes were originally calculated for this function. However, a growing body of research suggests that much higher intakes may also protect against cancer, autoimmune diseases, cardiovascular disease, diabetes, and other chronic illnesses.

Vitamin D is now regarded as a hormone by medical science because of its profound effects on most cells of the body at small doses. The light energy from sunlight causes a chemical reaction to occur in the cholesterol in our skin, converting cholesterol to vitamin D. The vitamin D is then transported to the liver and kidneys where it is made more active before it travels throughout the body, entering virtually every cell. Vitamin D makes its way to the nucleus of each body cell, where it instructs the genes to perform their necessary functions. Our bodies have evolved in such a complex way that, while most of our cells do not get exposed to sunlight, nature has given us this fantastic vitamin that carries the messages from the sun into the genes of our innermost cells. I regard it as the Universal Messenger that brings energy from the sun to our innermost soul.

Because vitamin D is transported to the liver and kidneys so that it can be made more active, the liver and the kidneys must be in good working order. In people with diabetes, the liver often has mild to moderate damage and the kidneys may have mild to severe damage. As a consequence of organ damage, the levels of active vitamin D may be extremely low, so it is essential for diabetics with weakened liver and kidney function to supplement with vitamin D.

The health of the liver is especially critical to the effective management of diabetes. The liver is a storage organ for the complex carbohydrate glycogen, which is broken down and released into the bloodstream as glucose. If the liver cells don't respond very well to insulin, they will start pumping out glucose, making the diabetes worse. Maintaining the health of the liver means avoiding toxic substances, such as alcohol, sugar, chemicals, preservatives that are added to foods, colorings and flavorings, pesticides, herbicides, and most drugs (including medications). Eliminating the toxic byproducts of the body's metabolism places enough stress on the liver without the organ also having to cope with the stresses of alcohol and other chemicals.

It is interesting to note that in some countries such as Australia, where people can be exposed to a lot of sunlight and therefore should have high levels of vitamin D in their bodies, there is actually an epidemic of vitamin D deficiency. This has come about for two main reasons. First, people are advised by public health authorities not to stay in the sun for too long for fear of the development of skin cancer, and to use sunblock to prevent ultraviolet light getting to the skin. Second, there has been a shift away from some of the fatty foods that are very high in vitamin D, in particular full cream cow's milk and its products.

VITAMIN D DEFICIENCY

Vitamin D deficiency can be quite serious, and may cause a number of very serious effects.

Rickets

In children, vitamin D deficiency can cause rickets, which results in skeletal deformities, bone pain, dental problems, impaired growth, and other symptoms. Although now rare, partially due to the availability of vitamin D-fortified milk, rickets may develop in children who do not regularly get enough sunlight, or children who cannot properly absorb vitamin D from the diet. Interestingly, infants and children who were given vitamin D supplements to prevent deficiency were less likely to get childhood onset (type 1) diabetes.

Osteomalacia

In adults, severe vitamin D deficiency can cause a condition called osteomalacia (soft bones) in adults, which results in muscular weakness in addition to weak bones. Osteomalacia may develop in adults with inadequate exposure to sunlight, those who have vitamin-D deficient diets, and individuals with decreased absorption of vitamin D.

Diabetes

It has been discovered that some newly diagnosed diabetics have relatively low levels of vitamin D. In fact, the higher the blood sugar levels, the lower the blood levels of vitamin D. This is a fascinating association. Indeed, vitamin D deficiency is commonly found in people with poor diabetes control. Unfortunately, as the deficiency worsens, so does blood sugar control. Therefore, diabetics should be screened regularly for vitamin D deficiency and should supplement with vitamin D, if necessary, under the care of a healthcare professional. The important message is that low blood levels of vitamin D should not be tolerated in any one, and more particularly in diabetics. Beyond this, it brings us to the point that *every* overweight person should have a fasting blood sugar and a vitamin D blood test. To me, these tests are just as important—in many cases, even more important—than going to the doctors and having your pulse and blood pressure checked. These facts are well-established in medical science and should be practiced routinely by all doctors.

Heart and Blood Vessel Diseases

Diseases of the arteries may occur as a result of a vitamin D deficiency. For people who have diabetes, it is these diseases of the arteries that are especially dangerous. Diseases of the arteries are made worse by diabetes and the use of insulin, and the presence of a vitamin D deficiency only exacerbates the problem. Low blood levels of vitamin D are also known to be associated with high blood pressure and a risk of heart disease. As diabetics are very susceptible to diseases of the heart and arteries, their vitamin D blood levels should be checked regularly. Because it has been found that vitamin D supplements alone may not have any influence on the development of heart disease, it is even more important for diabetics to obtain their vitamin D and other protective nutrients for the heart through dietary sources.

One of the most critical measures to take in diabetes management is the maintenance and protection of the pancreas and its insulin-producing cells. This can be achieved with vitamin D supplementation. The body produces a substance called C peptide that protects cells from damage, inflammation, and apoptosis or cell "suicide." It is important to have appropriate levels of C peptide in your system. The use of vitamin D supplements can actually increase significantly the blood levels of C peptide in diabetic patients. From this we can assume that vitamin D supplementation is again in the best interests of the diabetiç's health. And because it is a very safe vitamin, there is absolutely no reason it should not be given to all diabetics.

On the other hand, people who have diabetes may have cholesterol deposits in their arteries that can become calcified. Too much vitamin D can cause calcium to accumulate in these cholesterol deposits, making the hardening of the arteries even worse. Clearly, it is essential to maintain healthy levels of vitamin D and regularly monitor blood levels of the vitamin.

Immunity

On a number of occasions in this book I have mentioned that chronically high blood sugar levels can, in effect, poison the immune system. This problem is only exacerbated by chronic vitamin D deficiency, which can also compromise the immune system and may contribute to the onset of allergies and infections. Elderly people who have diabetes are extremely susceptible to infections, especially of the feet, kidneys, and lungs. Diabetics can also suffer more severely from infections that are easily fought off by people who do not have diabetes. For example, influenza in a diabetic could result in pneumonia, a very severe and life-threatening lung infection. However, supplementation with vitamin D can help protect against infections and illnesses. It has been shown in Japan that children supplemented with vitamin D during an influenza outbreak were less likely to get influenza, and if they did it wasn't so severe. Therefore, it makes sense to ensure that all diabetics, and in particular the elderly diabetic and the insulin-dependent diabetic, are given a vitamin D rich diet, sunlight, and appropriate vitamin D supplementation, especially at times before and during an influenza epidemic. I also recommend high doses of intravenous vitamin C for all diabetics who have suffered from severe influenza in the past, as well as supplementation with vitamin B complex and zinc.

Vitamin D deficiency may also be partially responsible for the development of autoimmune diseases, including diabetes, and supplementing with the vitamin may help prevent autoimmune diseases caused by viruses, vaccinations, and common allergies such as cow's milk allergy. There has been some suggestion that vitamin D deficiency may also increase risk of certain cancers including cancers of the breast, bowel, ovaries, pancreas and possibly cancer of the skin, although research in this area is ongoing. Deficiency or low intake of vitamin D may contribute to multiple sclerosis, rheumatoid arthritis, Parkinson's disease, Alzheimer's disease, and diseases of the arteries of the legs.

VITAMIN D DOSAGE

The amount of vitamin D that we need is called the dietary reference intake. It is the amount of vitamin D that we need to have in our diet, including supplements of vitamin D. It does not take into account how much time we spend in the sun getting our vitamin D from the sunlight. The recommended dietary intake for most adults is 600 international units (IU) per day, and for those over the age of seventy, 800 IU per day. The recommended upper level of vitamin D intake is generally no more than 4,000 IU daily in adults, and the usual maintenance dose is 1,000 IU per day. However, many nutritional and orthomolecular doctors have found that patients who are deficient in vitamin D will require at least 10,000 IU per day to correct a deficiency. If doses this high (or higher) are required, they should be prescribed by a properly qualified physician and monitored closely.

Vitamin D is measured in the blood. The amount of vitamin D in the blood reflects the amount of vitamin D produced in the skin as well as that from the diet. Vitamin D is stored in body tissues, so it is not that important to get sunlight every day but it is good if you can eat vitamin-rich foods as part of your diet. The exact level of vitamin D in the blood that is needed for good health is still controversial. If the level of vitamin D is below 25 nmol/L then rickets will occur in children and osteomalacia will occur in adults. A level of vitamin D above 40 nmol/L is okay for good health. However, many nutritional and orthomolecular doctors, as well as many orthodox doctors, believe that levels above 75 nmol/L are required for optimum health and the prevention of some of the cancers that occur in vitamin D deficiency.

Extremely high doses of vitamin D over a long period of time can be toxic. Vitamin D toxicity can cause extremely high blood levels of calcium, so an overdose of vitamin D produces the symptoms of an overload of calcium. These symptoms include nausea, vomiting, loss of appetite, and weakness. High blood levels of calcium may also result in calcium being deposited in the blood vessels, and the production of calcium oxalate kidney stones, as well as possible kidney damage. Thus, supplementation requires a balance—not too high a dose, not to low. Because vitamin D is a fat-soluble vitamin, people who are overweight and who carry a lot of fat in the abdominal area may also be storing vitamin D in this fat. Although blood tests may show that these individuals have low blood levels of vitamin D, these stores of vitamin D will be released from the fat into the bloodstream when there is significant weight loss. Therefore, blood tests for vitamin D and calcium levels may need to be done more frequently to make sure that the levels of these nutrients are not actually too high.

High doses of vitamin D are not generally required in treating people with diabetes. However if there is severe osteoporosis associated with the diabetes, vitamin D and calcium supplementation is important, in combination with supplements of important trace elements such as boron, zinc, manganese, and copper. One of the greatest strengtheners of bone is boron. Boron helps the male and female hormones to build up weakened bones.

Exposure to sunlight is still considered the most efficient way to maintain adequate vitamin D levels. Just ten to fifteen minutes of sunlight exposure a day—particularly on the hands, face, arms, back, or legs—is enough to satisfy the body's needs. Remember, however, that because exposure to UV rays is a risk factor for skin cancer, you should use sunscreen after that 10–15 minutes' exposure. More time in the sun or vitamin D supplementation may be necessary during the winter for people who live where daily sunlight is limited. Also, diabetics who have dark skin—even those who get regular exposure to sunlight—may not necessarily have good levels of vitamin D, and may need to improve their diet and take some supplements. The need for supplementation can be determined by a simple blood test.

Vitamin D occurs naturally in foods such as fortified milk, cheese, butter, eggs, fortified breakfast cereals, some meats, oysters, and fatty fish. Sardines (canned or fresh) are the richest source of vitamin D, followed by salmon, tuna, mackerel, catfish and eel. There are no vegetarian sources of vitamin D except for mushrooms that are not totally grown in the dark and that are exposed to ultraviolet light. These are an excellent source of vitamin D, almost as rich a source as sardines. The best sources of vitamin D—cod liver oil and halibut liver oil—were used by our mothers and grandmothers. Vitamin D from fish and possibly from the mushrooms can reduce complications of diabetes, including heart disease and immune failure. It can be very hard to get enough vitamin D from food sources alone. As a result, some people may need to take a vitamin D supplement in pill or capsule form.

CHAPTER 7

VITAMIN E COMPLEX

*In the 1950s the Shute brothers said vitamin E worked
against heart disease and cerebrovascular disease. They were
greeted with laughter. (Forty years later) the Harvard School
of Public Health showed that just 100 IU of vitamin E
per day decreased the death rate by 40 percent.*
—LINUS PAULING, PH.D.

Virtually every animal species requires vitamin E. Likes vitamins D and A, vitamin E is a fat-soluble vitamin. It is a
powerful antioxidant that protects fats and lipids from dangerous oxidation, which wreaks havoc on body cells and tissues. In
the nervous system, lipids protect cells and nerve fibers and aid
in the transmission of electrical impulses, the signals that cause
all muscles to move and the signals that send sensations such as
touch, heat, and pain from the skin to the brain. Without adequate amounts of vitamin E, the nervous system, brain, and many
other organs can be easily damaged by oxidation. Unfortunately,
by the time symptoms of vitamin E deficiency are seen or felt, a
severe deficiency has already occurred. Deficiency symptoms
include muscle weakness, incoordination, abnormal eye movements, and anemia caused when weakened cell membranes in red
blood cells rupture.

Vitamin E works very closely with vitamin C in protecting the
body's cells, membranes, and genetic material (DNA) against the

99

harmful effects of free radicals caused by medical drugs, toxins, chemicals, alcohol, radiation, and the effects of heavy metals such as lead, mercury, and arsenic. It also works with vitamin C and many other nutrients in maintaining a healthy immune system, which is so important for people with diabetes, who are so susceptible to reoccurring and possibly life-threatening infections.

Vitamin E is not simply a single compound, but consists of different forms called tocopherols and tocotrienols. Naturally occurring vitamin E actually has eight chemical forms: alpha-, beta-, gamma-, and delta-tocopherol and alpha-, beta-, gamma-, and delta-tocotrienol. These different forms have varying levels of biological activity, and as more research is being done, we are learning more about these activities.

The word "tocopherol" is taken from the Greek words for "to carry offspring" or "to bring forth childbirth." Vitamin E is found in wheat germ oil, which improves fertility in animals, so it is sometimes called the "fertility vitamin." We use whole-grain supplements and added vitamin E to sheep, cattle, and pig foods in Australia to improve fertility and production.

In 1931, Vogt-Moller of Denmark successfully treated habitual abortion in human females with wheat germ oil vitamin E. By 1939 he had treated several hundred women with a success rate of about 80 percent. In the 1930s doctors in England and Canada reported success in combating threatened abortion and pregnancy toxemias as well. Quite clearly vitamin E is of value in recurrent abortions.

The most natural state of vitamin E, which is a mixture of tocopherols and tocotrienols, is far superior to synthetic forms and is preferred to prevent industrialized societies major killer diseases heart disease, cancer, stroke and diabetes.

VITAMIN E AND DIABETES

As we have discussed, glucose provides energy that fuels all of the body's organ systems and their functions. When there is an excess of glucose in the blood, the sugar attaches itself to important proteins and enzymes that are necessary for the body's normal metabolic processes, and these proteins and enzymes malfunction. The hormone systems of the body are also seriously disturbed. The result is tissue damage and inflammation—the "biofire." Inflammation is the body's response to tissue damage, whether it is caused by trauma, surgery, radiation and radiotherapy, invading bacteria, or chemicals, including sugar and the body's own metabolic waste products. In this context, excess sugar has to be regarded as a foreign chemical that irritates the cells and tissues and results in inflammation. The more sugar is poured onto the biofire, the greater the low-grade chronic inflammation, especially in the deep fat tissues of the abdomen. It is these deep fat tissues where the most inflammation occurs in diabetes and metabolic syndrome, and it causes widespread damage to virtually every cell and tissue in the body. As an antioxidant, vitamin E is essential in helping to prevent inflammation and tissue damage. There is absolutely no doubt that low blood levels of vitamin E will result in the development of diabetes in a significant proportion of the population.

Vitamin E levels people who have type 2 diabetes are significantly lower than normal. This means that blood platelets are more likely to clump together and form mini-clots in the small blood vessels, especially those of the eye. This can lead to diabetic eye disease, known as diabetic retinopathy. If there is any suggestion that a diabetic's platelets are sticky, then vitamin E supplementation is essential to help prevent blindness. I have seen the use of vitamin E, vitamin C, and other nutrients important in the eye actually stop the development of diabetic retinopathy and in some fortunate cases actually cause it to reverse. Some patients have had the strength of their prescription glasses reduced and others in the early stages have found that their vision has improved to the point that spectacles are not always required. Of course the use of vitamin E in the prevention of diabetic retinopathy is imperative in people who have type 1 diabetes, as well. Vitamin E is a low-cost, readily available compound associated with few known side effects; thus, its use could have a dramatic socioeconomic impact if found to be efficacious in delaying the onset of diabetic retinopathy and/or nephropathy.

Vitamin E is a modest vasodilator that promotes collateral circulation and, consequently, offers great benefits to diabetes patients. Because of its anti-inflammatory properties and its ability to protect against damage from oxidative stress, vitamin E supplementation is necessary for diabetics who have heart disease, recurrent infections, inflammatory disorders, nerve and muscle degeneration, enlargement of the heart, and skin ulcers or wounds that do not heal. Diabetics with liver disease caused by alcohol abuse may also require vitamin E supplementation. In these situations, the vitamin E must be given with other nutrients for best effect. For example, zinc and vitamin C would be given along with vitamin E to treat skin ulcers and wounds that do not heal; selenium and coenzyme Q_{10} would be given for enlargement of the heart or heart failure.

Vitamin E reduces glycated hemoglobin (HbA1C), increases the antioxidant glutathione, and reduces blood sugar levels. Because the vitamin can lower blood glucose levels and, as a result, the amount of insulin required, there is less stress on the pancreas. Vitamin E can also help improve the levels of good cholesterol in the blood and combat the oxidation of cholesterol in the bloodstream, while at the same time lowering triglycerides—all of which help to decrease the risk of heart and blood vessel diseases. This powerhouse vitamin works synergistically with insulin to lower high blood pressure in people with diabetes. Together, all of these powerful actions of vitamin E can reduce the complications of diabetes. High doses of vitamin E, often referred to as pharmacological doses, not only improve the action of insulin in diabetics but also in healthy people.

Vitamin E has so many beneficial actions that, if it were a drug, it would be lauded as a miracle cure. To continue to ignore the important effects of vitamin E is tantamount to large-scale negligence. As it is not patented, it doesn't attract high profits; and a lack of high profits means no money from investors and no money for promotion and marketing to compete with inferior drugs.

DOSAGE

Despite the fact that the scientific studies prove the value of vitamin E in preventing and treating many diseases and conditions, and there has been a veritable explosion in antioxidant research since 1968, the RDA for vitamin E has, believe it or not, been decreased. Some governments such as the Australian government, have even attempted—unsuccessfully—to restrict the dosage in supplements.

The best dietary sources of vitamin E are whole grains, nuts, seeds and vegetable oils, and the recommended intake of vitamin E for adults is between 15 and 20 IU per day. However, in some disease conditions, vitamin E must be given in much higher doses for both prevention and treatment. The doses of vitamin E required to help prevent diabetes complications are far greater than the 15 to 20 IU per day typically recommended, up to between 1,000 and 3,000 IU per day. Doses of 1,000 to 1,500 IU per day can lower blood glucose levels, lessen the amount of insulin required needed to keep blood glucose levels within a healthy range, and decrease the stress on the pancreas to produce insulin, as well as improving cholesterol and triglycerides. These effects can be magnified with the addition of vitamin C. By adding a high dose of vitamin C, the requirement for vitamin E in treating diabetes can be reduced from 3,000 IU per day to between 500 and 1,000 IU per day. A combination of vitamin E at 1,000 mg per day plus nicotinamide at approximately 1,600 mg per day can reduce the requirements for insulin better than either alone, and they are both good for the heart and brain.

People with diabetes who also have narrowing of the arteries in the legs and suffer from pain in the calves (intermittent claudication), as well as those who are at risk of gangrene, would benefit from vitamin E supplementation. Intermittent claudication is now regarded as a reliable sign of peripheral arterial disease. A double-blind study has shown that it can be diminished by 66 percent with the use of vitamin E. The dosage administered is 1,600 mg per day and should be a natural form of vitamin E mixture or complex.

Even at the highest doses mentioned here vitamin E has been shown to be extremely safe and without side effects. The only caution is that it may increase the tendency to bleed in patients who are taking anticoagulants such as warfarin and aspirin. A person who is taking these medications and who plans to supplement with vitamin E should do so only under the supervision of a trained and experienced nutritional and orthomolecular physician.

One of the important things to remember with vitamin E supplementation is that the dose must be high enough and given for a relatively long period of time (anywhere from six to twelve months) to achieve its maximum benefit. Most of the scientific studies that have shown vitamin E to be effective have been conducted for at least four months.

CHAPTER 8

MINERALS AND
TRACE ELEMENTS

The physician is Nature's assistant.
—CLAUDIUS GALEN

It has been said that you command nature only by obeying her. I think this is a clear case of using what nature gave us to enable her to fight (or correct) the disease process in the gentlest of ways. Nature is truly a superpower!

It's very interesting to ponder on this because when you study most chronic and degenerative diseases, there is a very close relationship between these diseases (for example, cancer, heart disease, osteoporosis, stroke, arthritis, etc.) with multiple nutritional deficiencies. In other words, these serious and degenerative diseases may start with a genetic weakness combined with multiple deficiencies of minerals and trace elements.

It is very important that tests for these mineral levels be done in all diabetics, and in members of families in which diabetes is common. If this is not done, then the diabetic patient is at greater risk of developing the following problems:

• resistance to the body's insulin or the insulin given by injection

• very poor control of the diabetes

• a reduction in the pancreas's ability to secrete its own insulin

• high blood fats (cholesterol and triglycerides)

- disease of the very small arteries resulting in leg and foot ulcers and gangrene, which results in amputation, the surgical removal of the foot or leg.

- high blood pressure and heart failure

- abnormal rhythms and beating of the heart, and cardiac arrest

- kidney disease and kidney failure

- diseases of the eyes and blindness

- a tendency for the blood to clot and strokes (paralysis, inability to speak and possibly death)

CHROMIUM

Chromium is a trace mineral that plays a role in the metabolism of carbohydrates, fats, and proteins. It is essential in the function of insulin, as a component of a compound called glucose tolerance factor (GTF). GTF works together with insulin to open up channels in cell membranes that allow glucose enter the cells, where it can be used for energy. As glucose is taken up into cells, the blood glucose level drops. A low intake of chromium or an excessive loss of chromium results in poor sugar tolerance—the body just cannot handle sugars properly.

There are a variety of factors that cause or contribute to low levels of chromium in the body. Chromium is lost from the body as we age, and it is interesting to note that studies showing chromium depletion with age report the greatest decline being in the lungs. The importance of this is not fully understood, but we know that the lungs require a lot of sugar to produce the energy needed for the exchange of oxygen and carbon dioxide.

Chromium levels are also affected by mental and/or emotional stress, which is one of the reasons why stress management is so important in diabetes treatment. Additionally, the more sugar, refined carbohydrates, and alcohol we consume, the more chromium is washed out of the body via the kidneys. The use of cortisone tablets or creams can result in massive losses of chromium in the urine, as well. Thus, in a person with poorly controlled diabetes, who is already producing a high urine output to rid the body of excess sugar, chromium supplementation is essential when cortisone is taken. Because it appears that atherosclerosis and heart disease are also commonly associated with chromium, and we know people with diabetes are already more prone to heart disease, the importance of taking in adequate amounts of chromium cannot be overstated.

Certain tests can check for chromium levels in the body. The most common test is simply a blood test that measures chromium levels in blood plasma or red blood cells. Hair sample analysis may also be used to determine levels of minerals such as chromium, zinc, manganese, calcium, and iron. Tissue biopsy from the kidneys or liver is another option, although this procedure is risky and highly invasive, so it is not routinely performed.

Properly conducted clinical and scientific studies have proven the value of chromium in treating diabetes. A study published in 1998 by Dr. Hellerstein in *Nutrition Reviews* showed that a special form of chromium called chromium picolinate reduced fasting cholesterol, reduced HbA1C, reduced fasting plasma (blood) glucose, and fasting insulin levels dropped as well. These changes were all achieved over a relatively short period of four months, and all are statistically significant, which means they are all proven scientifically to be superior to a placebo. If the study had been conducted over a shorter period—as many drug studies are—the results may not have been so good. Drugs are generally fast acting. On the other hand, drugs have a multitude of harmful side effects because of their natural toxicity at typically-prescribed doses. Natural substances such as chromium may take longer to work than pharmaceutical products; however, when taken at therapeutic doses, supplements generally show no negative side effects and may, in fact, offer additional positive benefits. For example, chromium lowers blood glucose and its beneficial side effects are reduced cholesterol, triglycerides, and insulin requirements, plus more energy and no reactive hypo-glycemic symptoms. At the recommended doses, it is perfectly safe.

Type 2 diabetics and most type 1 diabetics respond well to chromium supplementation. People with diabetes who take chromium supplements will have an improvement in the action of insulin, which reduces the body's need for insulin and takes some of the stress off the pancreas. By increasing sensitivity to insulin, chromium helps diabetics reduce their blood sugar, fasting blood sugar, and HbA1C, as well as cholesterol and triglycerides. There is evidence that chromium may also help improve atheroscerosis, and it may mitigate or even partially reverse any nerve damage caused by chromium deficiency. For a small amount of an inexpensive mineral to be able to achieve all of this—and without harmful side effects—is almost a miracle.

In combination with chromium supplementation, exercise further increases insulin sensitivity and reduces insulin resistance, helping to push glucose into the cells of the muscles, heart, brain, liver, and kidneys. The benefits of an exercise program in addition to chromium supplementation will only help to improve blood sugar control in diabetes. Another important component of GTF is vitamin B_3, which was discussed in Chapter 5.

A particular type of yeast called brewer's yeast is a rich source of chromium. At one time, brewer's yeast (or nutritional yeast) was actually used in the nutritional treatment of diabetes, with some success. However, because many people with diabetes have or may develop an allergy or sensitivity to yeast, or more often, because of the odd taste, it is not currently recommended as a treatment for the disease, especially since chromium supplements are readily available.

Dosage

Chromium is required only in minute amounts in healthy people. For example, in babies and children the requirements are from 1 to 2 micrograms (mcg) per year of age; in adults, the recommended dose ranges from 25 to 50 micrograms per day. People who have diabetes need up to 500 micrograms per day; to correct a severe deficiency, the recommended dosage is 2,000 micrograms per day. It is important that the correct dose of chromium is established over the proper period of time, and need varies with different people. A qualified practitioner of orthomolecular-nutritional medicine is the best person for the job to ensure that pre-diabetic or diabetic patients are taking the optimal dose of chromium for their needs.

MAGNESIUM

It is well known that magnesium is necessary for proper nerve and muscle function, and that calcium is the all-important bone mineral. Well, like most things biological, it is not that simple. In fact, magnesium is as essential as calcium to bone structure and function. Studies have shown significant losses of magnesium from the bones in people with type 1 and type 2 diabetes, as well as some magnesium loss from the muscles. The use of insulin for the treatment of diabetes amplifies magnesium depletion. And because magnesium deficiency can actually increase one's chances of developing diabetes—as well as other conditions including heart disease, high blood pressure, and kidney stones—everyone should also be aware of the potential risks associated with low magnesium levels.

More than a third of people with diabetes have serious magnesium deficiencies and the rest have borderline levels that worsen over time. This occurs in all ages and with all forms of diabetes. The longer the diabetes has been present, the worse the magnesium deficiency. Magnesium deficiency is more profound in individuals whose diabetes is not well controlled, and who have to use higher doses of insulin and other diabetes medications to lower blood sugar. The body loses magnesium through urine, and because high blood glucose levels prompt a high output of urine in order to rid the body of excess sugar, poor blood sugar control means more magnesium is eliminated through urination. This creates a vicious cycle: high blood sugar leads to high urine output, which leads to magnesium depletion or deficiency that makes diabetes more difficult to control—and back to the beginning. Unfortunately, magnesium depletion never ceases entirely, even for people whose diabetes is well controlled. It appears that there will always be a loss of this magnificently powerful mineral. Therefore supplementation must be a lifelong habit.

One of the ways in which magnesium helps prevent cardiovascular and circulatory diseases appears to be its protective action against clotting. Small cell fragments within the blood called platelets are critical in stopping bleeding when there is an injury to a blood vessel. Platelets contain proteins on their surface that allow them to adhere to the site of injury in the blood vessel wall and seal the fissure. This is known as platelet aggregation, or clotting, and it is an important function. Unfortunately, without adequate levels of magnesium in the body, platelets can stick together and form clots where they are not needed. These clots can cut off circulation to the heart, brain, kidneys, eyes, or other vital organs, resulting in devastating consequences such as heart attacks, strokes, kidney failure, and blindness. Magnesium also aids in blood vessel dilation and lowers blood pressure, and it may help prevent against irregular heart rhythms—all of which are beneficial for cardiovascular health. Because diabetes increases one's risk of developing cardiovascular disease, supplementing with optimal levels of magnesium is an important preventive measure.

Magnesium supplementation, even without dietary changes, can help lower levels of "bad" LDL cholesterol, which tends to form plaques in arteries, as well as fats called triglycerides that circulate in the blood. Research has shown that high insulin levels increase LDL cholesterol and triglycerides; therefore, a person who has diabetes is at higher risk of developing cardiovascular illnesses such as atherosclerosis, heart attack, and stroke. However, high cholesterol and triglycerides can also predict diabetes by indicating insulin resistance even before a person develops the disease. In people who have diabetes, magnesium deficiency is a "double whammy": deficiency causes insulin resistance, and then the problem is compounded by high LDL cholesterol and triglycerides that interfere with insulin's action, making diabetes worse. Magnesium supplementation delivers a one-two punch that simultaneously improves the insulin response and lowers the levels of harmful blood fats.

Magnesium levels should be tested in every individual at risk of diabetes, and tests should be performed regularly depending on the person's medical history, nutritional status, weight, and family history. As magnesium is more important inside the body's cells than in the body's fluids, it is better to measure cellular levels of the mineral. Ideally, quantities of magnesium should be measured from the muscle, heart, or nerve cells; however, these samples are not easily obtained, and biopsies are rarely performed because of the danger involved. One day a handheld scanner may be available that shines a harmless beam into the brain or heart to obtain an instantaneous and inexpensive reading of the body's functional biochemistry. Until then, we can be satisfied that some of the cells in the blood give a fairly good indication of the amount of magnesium in the system overall. At this time, platelets and red blood cells appear to give relatively good measurements. Alternatively, your physician can do a "free ionized magnesium" test.

Dosage

Good dietary sources of magnesium include spinach and other dark leafy greens, almonds and cashews, soybeans, avocados, whole grains, beans, and fish such as salmon and halibut. However, the only sure way of maintaining optimal levels of magnesium is with supplementation and regular blood tests.

With magnesium in diabetes, prevention is better than cure.

Magnesium deficit or deficiency should be addressed immediately after a person is diagnosed with diabetes in order to prevent associated complications. At this time, there is no good evidence to show that diabetic retinopathy (eye disease) or diabetic nephropathy (kidney disease) can be stopped or reversed by magnesium alone. This is one reason why it is so important to take magnesium supplements in combination with other essential nutrients.

The recommended amount of magnesium intake is about 400 mg per day for adults. Some people will require more, including those who have diabetes or who are at risk of diabetes, particularly if tests show low platelet or red blood cell count; people who drink coffee, tea, and alcohol; and individuals who eat a nutritionally poor diet that includes little or no leafy greens. When there is a deficiency, the dose required to bring the body's magnesium levels back to the normal can range from 300 to 600 mg per day. Be aware that taking too much magnesium can cause side effects, including loose bowels or diarrhea, tiredness, and depression (although depression can also be associated with a lack of magnesium). One thing is for sure: an overdose of most nutrients is nothing as disastrous as an overdose of a drug.

MEASURING MINERAL MILLIGRAMS

A recommended dose of a mineral refers to the amount of the pure mineral itself, in its elemental form. Most supplement bottles clearly state the amount of the product per tablet. Sometimes, however, the front label can state a quantity of a mineral supplement including the chemical complex delivering it. This is not common, but can be misleading. Be sure to read the side label as well, where you will find a clear statement of how much of the actual mineral is contained in each tablet, or in two or three tablets. When in doubt, contact the manufacturer and ask. Reliable companies answer such inquiries promptly and completely.

The common forms of magnesium sold in pharmacies and health food stores are magnesium chelate, magnesium aspartate, and magnesium orotate. A healthcare professional can help you decide what form of magnesium is right for you. For people with diabetes who have existing cardiovascular disease, the magnesium of choice is magnesium orotate. This is because orotate carries magnesium most efficiently to the inside of the heart muscle cells, where it is most needed. The other advantage of magnesium orotate for patients taking statins to reduce cholesterol is that this form blocks some of the many harmful effects of statins—another win for nutrients over drugs.

ZINC

Zinc is another trace element that is required by every cell in the body. It is a cofactor, or "helper," that is involved in the synthesis and action of over 200 special proteins called enzymes that increase the rate of chemical reactions in the body. One of these enzymes, superoxide dismutase (SOD), acts as an antioxidant that helps to protect the body against a toxic substance called superoxide. Superoxide is an unstable, highly reactive compound that can damage body cells. As an enzyme, SOD acts quickly to remove superoxide from body tissues by breaking it down into oxygen and hydrogen peroxide. Two other trace elements, copper and manganese, are also important in the function of superoxide dismutase.

Besides its role as a component of superoxide dismutase, zinc has many other critical functions in the body, too. It is a necessary component of many hormones, including growth hormone and the sex hormones, and it is involved in the production and storage of insulin, as well as its release from the pancreas. Zinc is also important in the production, storage, and release of red and white blood cells, and in cell growth in general, so a high intake of zinc can be very helpful after times of emotional and physical stress, including a infection, trauma, and surgery. Zinc aids in proper function of the prostate and the kidneys, and adequate levels of the mineral are needed to help keep the hair and skin healthy.

A mild zinc deficiency is very common in modern Western civilizations, in which there is a high consumption of processed food. In general, nutritionally poor fad diets and anorexia will reduce one's intake of many essential minerals, including zinc, although even with adequate intake there is also the possibility that the body has a decreased ability to absorb zinc. The use and abuse of alcohol and diuretic drugs causes zinc to be washed out of the body, resulting in deficiency. Other common causes of zinc deficiency are vegetarianism, old age, diabetes, a high-fiber diet, chronic inflammatory disease and/or chronic infections, kidney dialysis, liver disease, celiac disease, chronic inflammatory bowel disease, chronic pancreatitis, and chronic diarrhea.

Symptoms of zinc deficiency include diarrhea, hair loss, skin conditions (such as eczema and acne), poor vision and night blindness, insomnia, mental or behavioral disturbances, and even psychiatric illness. It may cause loss of appetite and anorexia, which together can retard growth in young children and teenagers. Zinc deficiency can also delay sexual maturation in young people. People who have zinc deficiency may develop inflammatory bowel disorders and malabsorption syndrome, in which foods are not properly absorbed into the body from the gut. This aggravates any disease condition, as it makes already existing deficiencies even worse. It is interesting to note that zinc deficiency can reduce the senses of smell and taste, which further aggravates loss of appetite and anorexia and, as a result, exacerbates zinc deficiency.

The immune system is dependent on zinc to function properly. Zinc is essential to the activity of white blood cells in fighting illnesses and infections. It is also important in hormones related to the immune system function, including insulin, which ensures that glucose can enter the white blood cells to give them the energy necessary to fight invaders. There is evidence that zinc has a direct killing activity on viruses, as well, such as by binding onto the virus that causes the common cold.

Because deficiency weakens the immune system, a person who is not getting enough zinc might suffer from numerous infections, including infections of the throat, sinuses, lungs, skin, and urinary tract. In addition, poor wound healing and slow recovery from infection may be partially the result of zinc deficiency. The use of zinc supplements can dramatically reverse poor immune function. This is particularly important for people who have diabetes, because they are typically more prone to infection. A word of caution, however: very high doses of zinc can actually impair the immune system, so it is extremely important to make sure that the dose is optimal—high enough for the desired effect without being too high.

In men, zinc deficiency may cause the prostate gland to swell, resulting in the need for medications and/or surgery. Infertility may also result from deficiency, due to a reduction in the number of sperm, an increase in abnormal sperm, and a lack of sperm activity. Because zinc is important in the production of male sex hormones, low levels of the mineral may reduce the production of testosterone. This is compounded by erectile dysfunction, another common problem in men with diabetes that can result from damage to nerves and blood vessels caused by the disease. These problems can often be helped with a correct dose of zinc and adjustments to diet. There is also some evidence that deficiency may cause of infertility in women, so a trial of zinc supplementation may be worthwhile for infertile couples before they embark on measures such as in vitro fertilization (IVF). The other nutrient that infertile couples should try before resorting to IVF is vitamin C, taken at 1,000 mg a day (each) for 3 to 6 months.

Because pregnancy increases the body's requirements for zinc, and because diabetes itself may cause zinc deficiency, women who develop gestational diabetes should be particularly concerned about getting adequate amounts zinc. In fact, zinc may help prevent diabetes during pregnancy, so women who are pregnant or who may become pregnant should ensure that they are taking in adequate levels of the mineral. Zinc is very important for the development of the baby; deficiency during pregnancy may result in premature birth, as well as low birth weight or growth retardation. Some research has suggested that there is a link between zinc deficiency and the development during pregnancy of a dangerous condition called pre-eclampsia. Symptoms of pre-eclampsia include fluid retention, high blood pressure, and excess protein in the urine (proteinuria). Because zinc is so crucial for a healthy pregnancy—and a healthy baby—it may be just as important for pregnant woman to take zinc as it is for her to take iron and a daily multivitamin.

One of the common signs of zinc deficiency is the presence of white spots on the fingernails. However this sign is not a very good indicator of the overall levels of zinc in the body. One of the best tests for zinc is to measure the amount of zinc in the white blood cells.

Dosage

Zinc is found in high concentrations in fish and red meat. It also is found in oysters and other shellfish, and whole cereal grains. Adults can safely supplement with zinc in addition to a good diet. However, for a patient with diabetes, higher doses of zinc are necessary for the reasons outline above. The doses of zinc for men may need to be up to 60 mg per day and, for women, to 45 mg per day. Doses of 100 mg per day for short periods may necessary for people with severe deficiencies.

Taking too much zinc can cause nausea. This is one of the first signs of an excessive intake. Prolonged use of zinc at 150 mg or more per day can displace copper from the body, and copper deficiency anemia may occur. The immune system may become compromised, resulting in more infections, principally of the airways and urinary tract. In addition to anemia, low levels of copper in the system caused by too much zinc can reduce levels of "good" HDL cholesterol, which would place a person with diabetes at a greater risk of heart disease.

Zinc should always be taken on an empty stomach. Do not take zinc close to mealtimes, especially when a meal contains cereal grains, as there are substances in grains such as wheat, barley, rye, and oats that bind onto zinc and prevent its absorption in the body. Also, for maximum absorption, it is best to leave a good amount of time between taking zinc and other mineral supplements, including calcium, magnesium, and iron.

VANADIUM

The trace mineral vanadium appears to have a role in regulating glucose metabolism and reducing blood sugar levels. Vanadium has a very similar action to insulin. It has been shown to stimulate the uptake of glucose into cells, and it increases the conversion of glucose to its storage form, glycogen, which acts as an energy reserve that can be tapped if the body has a sudden demand for glucose. At the same time, vanadium helps prevent the body from using protein components called amino acids as an energy supply when glucose runs low. Proteins are essential building blocks for muscles, bone, skin, hair, and other tissues; thus, it is important for proteins to be available for these functions, rather than being used for energy. Vanadium also provides the benefit of improving the metabolism of glucose in fat cells and skeletal muscle, and decreasing blood cholesterol, particularly the "bad" LDL cholesterol.

The form of vanadium used in treating type 2 diabetes is vanadyl sulfate. It is not proven scientifically whether vanadium is of any value in type 1 diabetes. However, it appears that it is able to actually reduce the needs for insulin, which is a huge advantage. It also reduces the harmful side effects of high insulin dosages in children and type 1 diabetics, so its use in type 1 is strongly recommended. Consult your physician about dosage.

CALCIUM

We all know that calcium is very important for the development of bones and teeth, as well as for nervous system function. We also know that with advancing age, calcium and other minerals are lost from bone, decreasing bone density and increasing the risk of fractures. The medical term for loss of bone density is *osteoporosis,* and it can have serious complications such as fractures of the hip and back that may occur even if there is no injury or trauma.

It is now becoming clear that people who have diabetes—especially individuals whose diabetes is not well controlled—have an increased risk of developing osteoporosis. Research suggests that patients with type 1 diabetes are at greater risk of osteoporosis than those with type 2 diabetes, although postmenopausal women who have type 2 diabetes also show an elevated risk. The mechanisms of diabetes-related osteoporosis are still not entirely clear, but it does seem that people who have diabetes show a tendency for calcium to be lost from the body through the urine. Combined with deficiencies of other minerals important to bone health, including zinc and magnesium, the loss of calcium from the body causes bones to become weak and prone to fractures. Nutrient-poor diets loaded with sugar and white flour products; sodium; excessive protein; excessive cereal grains; and coffee, tea, and other caffeinated beverages are detrimental to bone health, as well as to overall health.

The minerals that we discuss in this book are all related to one another directly or indirectly in terms of health and diabetes. This is not a book about the treatment of osteoporosis, but it is important that diabetic patients recognize the fact that they are at risk of this serious bone disease, and prevention is key. Calcium works with many other nutrients—including magnesium, vitamin K, and vitamin D—to build and preserve bone health. Some of these nutrients aid calcium absorption, while others prevent it. Vitamin D is absolutely essential for the absorption of calcium from the intestine into the bloodstream and helps maintain blood levels of calcium.

As you can see, diabetes is not just a blood-sugar disorder. It is a multi-organ disease and virtually no organ, tissue, or cell in the body is unaffected. Why the kidneys lose calcium and other minerals essential to bone health is unclear, but every patient must be aware of the risks of nutrient deficiencies.

POTASSIUM

Potassium is an essential mineral for nervous system function and muscle contractions, including contractions of the heart muscle. It also plays an important role in the body's acid-base balance, and because people who have diabetes tend to experience higher-than-normal levels of acid (see diabetic ketoacidosis on page 10), potassium is particularly crucial to good health. Balancing acids and bases in the body is necessary to maintain hydration and to keep organs such as the kidneys and the heart, as well as nerves and muscle, functioning properly. Additionally, potassium improves insulin sensitivity in people who have diabetes, and it is also aids the body in storing glucose as glycogen, which can be used later for energy.

Potassium deficiency may occur in people with diabetes who use insulin, as well as those who take diuretics to control hypertension (which, as we know, often occurs with type 2 diabetes in particular). As diuretics rid excess fluids from the body, important nutrients are also flushed out through urination. Other causes of deficiency include poor absorption of the mineral, as well as factors that cause the body to lose potassium, such as prolonged exercise and/or excessive sweating, and a diet high in sodium.

Intense exercise is another potential culprit of low potassium levels. Of course, exercise is beneficial for people who have diabetes because it improves insulin sensitivity and glucose metabolism. However, exercising too hard and for too long causes the body to lose potassium from the muscles, and some amount of the mineral is lost in sweat. Anyone who makes regular, intense exercise a part of his or her daily routine should guard against losing too much potassium, but diabetics must be particularly careful because of other factors that can cause low potassium, such as insulin shots and possibly the use of diuretics.

More than 90 percent of the body's potassium is held inside the cells, while most of the sodium in the body is pumped out of the cells. If too much sodium remains within the cells, they swell up and malfunction. Thus, potassium deficiency will impair the function of cells in the brain, nervous system, and heart. Diabetics who also have kidney disease are at greater risk.

Symptoms of potassium deficiency include fatigue, irritability, muscle weakness and problems with muscle coordination, poor conduction of nerve impulses, and abnormal heart rhythms. A blood test to determine the amount of potassium inside the red blood cells is the best way of monitoring potassium levels.

Dosage

Low potassium in people with diabetes is frequently overlooked, but it is one of the easiest problems to remedy with simple dietary changes. Good sources of potassium include all meats, some types of fish, and many fruits and vegetables. Dairy products are also typically good food sources of the mineral. Interestingly, scientific studies have shown that increasing the intake of fruit and vegetables by two to three portions per day can decrease hypertension and associated risks, such as stroke. It may be that fruits and vegetables reduce blood pressure because of their potassium content, or it may be that the bioflavonoids in fruits and vegetables strengthen the walls of the arteries. Whatever the cause of these wonderful benefits, it is an excellent reason for recommending more of nature's whole foods in the diet.

Potassium is obviously a critical component of good health, but taking supplements has the potential for overdose. Therefore, it is best to consult a qualified healthcare professional who can monitor potassium levels and help you manage any abnormalities.

As discussed above, many diabetics also have high blood pressure, which may be aggravated by low potassium in the system, particularly when sodium intake from the diet is much greater than potassium intake. One of the best measures for addressing hypertension is to begin by cutting back on salt in the diet and, at the same time, adding several more servings of fruits and vegetables. Potassium supplements that provide 3 to 5 g of potassium per day may be required to reduce blood pressure. Supplements are in the form of potassium salts, including potassium chelate, potassium aspartate, potassium citrate, potassium chloride, potassium bicarbonate, and potassium orotate. If you will be supplementing with potassium, it is essential to discuss with your healthcare provider which form of the mineral will work best for you. It takes only a few weeks for potassium to reduce high blood pressure and it works very well in the elderly who may not be able to take medications to lower blood pressure.

Be aware that taking in too much potassium from can cause side effects, including nausea, vomiting, and diarrhea, so supplementation should be undertaken only under the advice and guidance of a qualified healthcare provider. Potassium from dietary sources typically will not cause these problems, although people with kidney disease may need to restrict their intake of potassium. It is interesting to note that most kidney disease will respond to added vitamin C (1 to 4 g), which also may help to lower blood pressure and cholesterol. If kidney disease improves with the use of vitamin C, then a higher dose of supplemental potassium is possible. Potassium should not be given to patients with heart disease who are taking digitalis, certain diuretics, and some blood pressure lowering drugs.

MANGANESE

Like zinc, manganese functions in many enzyme systems, including those involved in energy production, thyroid function, immunity, and blood sugar control. And like zinc, it is a component of the superoxide dismutase (SOD), so it is an important part of the body's antioxidant defense mechanisms. Manganese also works with vitamin K in blood clotting. In animals, a deficiency of manganese can result in diabetes and even the failure of the pancreas to develop properly. In humans, supplementation with manganese has been shown to improve diabetes control, even in patients who do not respond well to insulin treatment. There is no doubt that adequate levels of manganese are helpful in the treatment of diabetes.

Manganese deficiency in animals can cause slow or inadequate growth and impaired fertility. If a deficiency occurs during pregnancy, the offspring suffer from a lack of balance and coordination caused by the failure of the inner ear to develop properly. Manganese deficiency can also cause problems with carbohydrate and fat metabolism and even result in defects of the skeleton. In humans, manganese deficiency does not often produce clearly recognizable symptoms, but some problems do exist, including skin rashes, abnormal bone growth, reduced "good" HDL cholesterol, poor hair and nail growth, and even the loss of the normal coloring or pigment in the hair.

Dosage

Dietary sources of manganese include dark green leafy vegetables, such as mustard greens and collard greens; Brazil nuts, almonds, and pecans; whole grains like buckwheat, rye, and barley; and pineapples. As a supplement, the mineral is available in forms called manganese chelate and manganese picolinate. Most people will need to take about 5 mg per day, but individuals who have diabetes may require as much as 15 mg per day. If a diabetic patient develops an ulcer, has an accident with trauma to large areas of tissue, or undergoes surgery, it would be prudent to supplement the patient with substantial doses of zinc and manganese to ensure that the inflammatory response to tissue injury is rapidly followed by the healing response. Copper, which is another trace element, is equally important in the inflammatory response and healing, so supplementing with copper may also be useful in these circumstances.

Manganese has a very low level of toxicity, so the supplements that are available are extremely safe. A condition known as "manganese madness" has been known to occur, but this typically has affected people who are in an environment that has been heavily polluted due to manganese mining.

SELENIUM

Selenium is a trace mineral required in very small doses in the body. As a component of the enzyme glutathione peroxidase, selenium is a powerful antioxidant. It is important in the detoxification of rancid fats in the body called lipid peroxides. It also protects against the harmful effects of hydrogen peroxide (bleach), which is produced during metabolism. These antioxidant actions are strengthened when selenium works together with vitamin E.

Selenium and glutathione peroxidase help to support eye health by protecting against oxidation of the lens and retina. The lens of the eye is at a high risk of oxidation because of its continued exposure to light; cataracts may form as a result. Oxygen damage can also damage the retina of the eye. This type of damage is called age-related macular degeneration and, as the name suggests, it grows steadily worse with age. Because people who have diabetes are at greater risk of developing certain diseases of the eye, it is particularly important for these individuals to take in adequate levels of selenium to protect against eye problems.

Some studies have suggested that selenium also enhances immunity through its antioxidant action. Glutathione peroxidase is found in high concentration in white blood cells called lymphocytes, which provide a line of defense against bacteria, viruses, and other foreign invaders. Selenium can help stimulate the activity of white blood cells and, potentially, protect these important immune cells against harmful oxidation. It also stimulates the production of antibodies in the blood to fight infections.

We also know that selenium has a role in maintaining normal heart rhythm and function, and it eases blood flow by reducing the "stickiness" of blood platelets. In this way, selenium has an effect similar to that of aspirin, without the toxicity. Also, higher blood levels of selenium seem to have a protective effect when it comes to hypertension—that is, higher levels of selenium may help lower the blood pressure.

Selenium is present in cell nuclei, which contain our genetic material. Because it appears that selenium helps prevent damaged DNA molecules from reproducing, we can see how the mineral may have a role in protecting our genes. Selenium also has a powerful effect on suppressing the processes that cause cancer. It also counteracts many of the effects of chemical allergies and sensitivities.

Selenium is found largely in soil, and plant foods are a major dietary source of the mineral in most countries. The content of selenium in foods depends on the selenium content of the soil where plants are grown or animals are raised. Many soils in the United States, Australia, and New Zealand are very poor in their selenium content; thus, foods grown in the soil and animals raised on the land will have lower selenium levels. Cattle and sheep raised on selenium-poor lands may be infertile, and show poor development and white muscle disease. Selenium is also lost in the cooking process. Severe stress and over-exercising are two other possible causes of selenium deficiency.

Because selenium aids in the production of thyroid hormone, which determines the rate of metabolism, it is a particularly important mineral for people with diabetes or metabolic syndrome. While blood levels of selenium in people who have diabetes are generally regarded as normal, the amount of selenium in red blood cells may be low, especially in insulin-dependent diabetics. Selenium deficiency in people with diabetes may be the result of undiagnosed celiac disease. In fact, celiac disease should be suspected in any diabetic who exhibits a deficiency of any trace mineral. If celiac disease is not present, then a non-celiac gluten enteropathy (allergy to wheat gluten) is most likely, and gluten-containing grains must come out of the diet. No matter what the cause of the deficiency, selenium supplementation is essential to help prevent the development of diabetic neuropathy.

There is a link between selenium deficiency and an increased risk of cardiovascular problems, including atherosclerosis (hardening of the arteries), high blood pressure, and heart attacks. These three conditions are all known complications of metabolic syndrome and diabetes. A severe selenium deficiency combined with other nutritional deficiencies may even cause a gross enlargement of the heart called cardiomyopathy, which can lead to heart failure and possibly the need for heart transplant surgery.

Because selenium is important to immune system function, deficiency can cause increased susceptibility to infections. Low levels of selenium may result in the inability of white blood cells to attack invading bacteria and viruses, as well as the failure of "killer cells" of the immune system to destroy them. Some typically harmless viruses can actually become highly virulent if the body is deficient in multiple nutrients, including selenium, vitamin E, zinc, or vitamin C. This is probably the case with most infections. One good example is Coxsackie virus B_3, which is harmless unless the individual carrying the disease is deficient in selenium and vitamin E. Deficiencies cause a change in the virus genes and it will attack the heart.

Selenium may be low in patients who have inflammation of the pancreas, or pancreatitis, which has the potential to become quite serious. Symptoms of pancreatitis include abdominal pain, digestive problems, and weight loss. As we know, the pancreas manufactures and secretes insulin, so maintaining healthy pancreatic function is essential for everyone, and especially for people who are at risk of diabetes. Supplementing with selenium has been shown to reduce the pain and the frequency of attacks in patients with chronic pancreatitis. High-dose intravenous selenium is an effective treatment for acute pancreatitis, resulting in a significant reduction of complications and death. Orthodox medicine has very little to offer patients who suffer from acute pancreatitis apart from the maintenance of intravenous fluids.

The liver is involved in the production of glucose, so keeping this organ healthy is imperative in people who have diabetes or who are at risk of developing the disease. Alcohol and tobacco use can damage the liver and, as a result, impair its ability to maintain blood glucose levels within a normal range. Moreover, both alcohol and tobacco appear to deplete selenium in the liver, which only worsens the problem. Selenium supplementation may help to improve liver function.

Studies have also focused on selenium's role in sperm motility and its possible usefulness in supporting fertility in men. There is an increased likelihood of infertility in men who have diabetes, and selenium deficiency may exacerbate this problem. Selenium deficiency is associated with a reduced level of the male sex hormone testosterone, a decrease in the mobility of sperm, and an increase in the number of abnormal sperm. Supplementing with selenium may help to improve fertility, particularly in combination with other nutrients, including vitamin E, vitamin C, zinc, fish oil, and vitamin B-complex.

Dosage

Selenium is found in organ meats and Brazil nuts. Many vegetables and grains contain selenium, but only if they are grown in soil with a high content of selenium. Garlic is also a rich source of selenium if the soil contains appropriate levels of the mineral.

Selenium can become toxic; however, in the correct dose and form it is essential for life. The Japanese diet of fish and other seafoods, including seaweed, is extremely high in selenium and this may be one reason for the very low incidence of cancer in Japanese people.

The organic form of selenium is safest. Organic selenium is known as selenomethionine. While the Japanese diet may provide up to 800 mcg (micrograms) of selenium per day, clinical trials have shown that using 400 mcg per day over several years is reasonably safe. The safe upper limit dose of selenium over a long period is considered to be 200 mcg per day. A qualified healthcare professional should help you determine your need for this mineral.

CHAPTER 9

OTHER NUTRIENTS

The best doctor gives the least medicines.
—BENJAMIN FRANKLIN

There is no such thing as monotherapy for diabetes. No single pill; no single injection; no single drug; and no single nutrient. As any sports player will tell you, it takes the whole team to win.

OMEGA-3 FISH OILS

I can't really answer this question about whether or not fish get heart disease and diabetes. I doubt if they do. My grandmother taught me that fish were very smart because they were always in schools, and that if I ate fish I would be very smart. My grandmother was pretty smart herself, despite not having a formal education. Big fish eat smaller fish, so I guess that makes them nutritionally smart. It's almost the perfect diet—a fresh, whole food without additives.

These days we can purchase fish oil in capsules. Back in my grandmother's day, the only fish oil that was available was the nasty tasting cod-liver oil that she used for preventing and treating coughs and colds. We now know that the oil in the fish is good for the brain and the vitamin A and D in the cod liver oil is good for the immune system.

The active ingredients in fish oil are the omega-3 fatty acids called eicosapentaenoic acid (EPA) and docosahexaenoic acid (DHA). Sorry about those long ten-dollar chemical names, but they really are important. These essential fatty acids, or EFAs, are found in the cell membranes of virtually every cell in the body. They keep the membranes structurally sound and help to maintain the shape of the cell. They also play a very important role in reducing inflammation and helping to resolve inflammatory reactions. Using an oil to suppress a fire seems like an unusual concept, except in this case we are attempting to quench the "biofire" of inflammation.

We now know that the oil in the fish is good for the brain, and the vitamin A and D in cod liver oil is good for the immune system. Science has also shown us that fish oil plays an important role in the prevention of some cancers, heart disease, many skin disorders, and some brain diseases and mental conditions including depression and schizophrenia. It also plays a role in slowing the aging process and may help to slow down the progression of some of the symptoms of Alzheimer's disease.

The omega-3 essential fatty acids in fish oils reduce the stickiness and thickness of the blood in people who have diabetes. This is important because it helps to reduce the risk of blood clots in the arteries and, therefore, lowers the risk of a heart attack or stroke. The other benefit of omega-3 is that if small clots do form, the fatty acid helps to break these small clots down more efficiently. Fish oils also reduce blood pressure and triglycerides.

In the past, the only fish oil available was the less-than-tasty cod-liver oil used for preventing and treating coughs and colds. These days we can purchase fish oil in capsules. The oil is obtained from the tissues and intestines of oily fish. However, the best way to consume fish oil is to eat fish. The safest fish to eat are the small fish, such as sardines and herring. These fish obtain their omega-3 fatty acids from algae in the sea. Larger fish—for example, tuna, swordfish, and shark—contain the omega-3 but they also contain toxins such as dioxin, PCBs, and heavy metals including mercury. These larger fish are higher up the food chain and are less safe to consume because of these contaminants.

The recommended dose of fish oil for diabetic patients with heart disease is 1 g to 2 g per day in capsule form. It is also recommended that the diabetic patient eat two to three meals of fish per week. However, the dose of fish oil should not exceed 4 g daily. If too much fish oil is consumed, the blood can become very thin and easy bruising and a tendency to bleeding can occur. This is particularly dangerous if the patient suffers from trauma or has to undergo surgery. This tendency to bleed may also increase the risk of a bleeding episode, or stroke, in the brain. Doses of fish oil higher than 5 g a day actually increase the blood sugar levels and raise bad cholesterol, especially in diabetics who are obese.

A simple blood test can determine if cells lack of omega-3 EFAs. If this is the case and the diabetic patient is also suffering from depression, the depressed mood may improve with fish oil supplements and an increased intake of fish in the diet.

INOSITOL AND MYOINOSITOL

The vitamin-like substance inositol is a very important component of all cell membranes. It also helps to break down and remove fat from the liver and other cells, and appears to play a role in the function of some neurotransmitters and messenger molecules, which can aid in depression. Inositol may help mitigate diabetic neuropathy, a nerve disease that is a complication of long-term diabetes. In people with diabetes, the nerves tend to lose inositol; thus, replacement may help to improve nervous system function.

Early medical studies with the substance inositol were not very convincing of its efficacy. However, more recent studies using myoinositol, which is converted from inositol in muscles, are more promising. Myoinositol given to diabetics over a period of two weeks at a dose of 500 mg twice daily was shown to produce significant improvement in nerve function. A diet high in inositol assists in the functioning of damaged nerves.

Inositol is found in foods as a component of fiber; food sources include nuts, seeds, legumes, and citrus fruits. It is bound up in the fiber component of food as a substance known as phytic acid or inositol hexaphosphate—a substance believed, with some evidence, to have very strong anti-cancer effects.

CARNITINE

Carnitine is produced from an amino acid called lysine. As its name implies, carnitine comes from meat. It is also found in dairy foods. Its function is to carry fatty acids into the cell mitochondria, which is where the fatty acids are used to produce energy.

Carnitine is in short supply in patients with type 2 diabetes who have complications such as retinopathy (eye disease), neuropathy (nerve disease), and high cholesterol, as well as in those who are treated with insulin. When patients who have type 2 diabetes are given carnitine supplements, the uptake of glucose from the bloodstream and into the cells is improved. If carnitine is given on a daily basis for four to six months, cholesterol and blood fats are significantly reduced. Carnitine is therefore essential for diabetic patients who have high blood fats.

Another form of carnitine, known as acetyl-l-carnitine, also benefits patients with diabetic neuropathy. Acetyl-L-carnitine significantly relieves the pain, numbness, and "pins and needles" sensations that are symptoms of neuropathy. The dosage is 500 mg twice daily. Interestingly, acetyl-L-carnitine enhances the activity of other antioxidants in the body and protects cells, including nerve cells, against free radical damage. The important thing to remember here is that acetyl-L-carnitine should be used to prevent diabetic neuropathy in patients who are at risk.

ALPHA-LIPOIC ACID

Alpha-lipoic acid (ALA) aids in glucose uptake into body cells, helps improve metabolism in people with diabetes, and acts as an antioxidant that can reduce the oxidative stress in diabetes. It also reduces a harmful acid known as lactic acid in the blood.

ALA has a beneficial action in peripheral neuropathy, reducing the pain, numbness, and abnormal sensations that are associated with this complication of diabetes. It has been given daily as an intravenous injection but it can also be given orally at 600 mg three times a day. If the nerves to the heart have been affected by neuropathy and the heart is suffering as a consequence, the use of oral alpha-lipoic acid is also recommended.

EVENING PRIMROSE OIL

I have a little saying that helps people remember where their important health-giving oils come from: omega-6 from the sticks (land plants) and omega-3 from the sea (fish oils). There are one or two exceptions to this—the most important being linseed oil, a land plant oil from the sticks that contains mostly omega-3.

The reason that I have included evening primrose oil in this book is that people with diabetes (type 1 diabetes in particular) often have low levels of a substance called gamma linolenic acid (GLA). Primrose oil is a rich source of GLA, and up to 6 g per day of evening primrose oil has been shown to improve the symptoms diabetic neuropathy. Better still, rather than waiting for neuropathy to develop, with its pain and troublesome skin sensations, it would make sense to test for GLA levels and supplement in the very early stages of the disease (as is the case with most of the nutrients discussed in this book). However, please also remember that most of the complications and problems with diabetes are not caused by the lack of one nutrient alone or a single food.

Finally, men who have diabetes often experience difficulty

achieving or maintaining and erection. The GLA in evening primrose oil is converted in the body to another compound called
DGLA that is then converted to a prostaglandin called PGE1.
PGE1 is marketed as a drug that can be injected into the penis,
or inserted into the hole at the head of the penis. Taking a single
dose of evening primrose oil will not enable a male to instantly
achieve an erection, nor will taking massive doses be effective.
However, over a period of months, the ingestion orally of primrose oil at modest doses of 1 to 2 g per day may cause a buildup
of PGE1 that can help to alleviate impotence. It certainly won't
do any harm. I would recommend the same dose of fish oil be
consumed. Another proven treatment for this problem is the
long-term use of panax ginseng at a dose of 1 g to 2 g per day.

FLAVONES

Flavones are special antioxidants found in many healthy foods,
including quercetin in onions, lycopene in tomato sauce, and
bioflavonoids in citrus fruits. Antioxidants are especially important for people with diabetes, whose cells, tissues, and organs suffer damage from oxidative stress. Scientific studies have shown
that the flavones such as quercetin and lycopene can protect
against oxidative damage to DNA. Also, rutin and quercetin
can reduce sugar coating that poisons hemoglobin in red blood
cells. Hemoglobin transports oxygen throughout the body, and
flavones makes this process more efficient. Up to 2 g per day of
special bioflavonoids can lessen the damage that occurs to very
small blood vessels. This reduces the amount of fluid leaking out
of the blood vessels and damaging the nerves, eyes, and kidneys.

CHAPTER 10

HERBAL MEDICINES

*What is a weed? A plant whose virtues
have not been discovered.*
—EMERSON

Long before there were any drugs, or any food supplements,
there were herbs and spices. Today, when we investigate
medicinal plants, we are, in a way, reinventing the wheel. The
plants have always been there. What is new is our ever-increasing knowledge of their many benefits.

PORTULACA (D-PURSLANE)

Portulaca (D-Purslane) is an extract of the herb Portulaca (D-Purslane) with a long tradition of application in medicine. Its use
dates back to ancient Egypt and there are records that it was used
medicinally in Crete and Greece. It has also been used as a tea
for sore throats and a treatment for earaches. In the near East,
South America, and Mexico it has been valued for its effects in
the treatment of diabetes.

Portulaca (D-Purslane) works in three ways to help control
blood sugar levels in the body: it improves the sensitivity of
cells to insulin, it reduces the amount of glucose that is absorbed
from the intestine into the bloodstream, and it increases the
uptake of glucose from the blood and into the cells. The other

very important feature of D-Purslane is that it may also help to reduce HbA1C, which is a long-term blood test marker for blood glucose control. A high HbA1C means you have an increased risk for developing heart and blood vessel disorders. Portulaca (D-Purslane) has been shown scientifically to reduce HbA1C levels. The levels are in line with the target recommended by the American College of Endocrinology. This means that it is important in the long-term management of diabetes. Additionally, D-Purslane can help prevent diabetes if it is used as in intervention when high blood sugar levels are first detected. It is therefore a very useful natural herbal medicine and should be considered for use in all pre-diabetics and diabetics in conjunction with diet, exercise, vitamin and mineral supplementation, and other therapies when necessary.

Drugs that are currently used to treat diabetes called glitazones act on a part of the cell membrane called the PParGamma receptor. These drugs stimulate this receptor to improve the sensitivity of the cell to insulin. This means that these drugs aid insulin in working more efficiently, and pump more sugar into the cell to be used as energy. However these drugs also stimulate the PParGamma receptor to pump more fatty acids into the cell and promote weight gain. Portulaca (D-Purslane) on the other hand, is more selective in this stimulation and does not promote weight gain.

GARLIC: VINYLDITHIINS AND DISULFIDES (V & D SULFIDES)

We all know the wonderful value of garlic as an herb that is used in many delicious recipes from around the world. It has a very pungent odor when cut but imparts a fantastic flavor dimension in cooking. For many years it has been claimed that garlic has tremendous medicinal properties but there has been a lot of scientific controversy over its value as a treatment. However recent evidence shows that garlic extracts, if they are properly prepared, do have very powerful effects . Specially prepared extracts of garlic contain V & D sulfides that can balance the blood fats and cholesterol and can also reduce the oxidation of the fats in the blood. Most diabetics, pre-diabetics, and people with the metabolic syndrome have a disturbance in the fats in their blood. This includes high levels of cholesterol and triglycerides, not only in the bloodstream but also in their fat cells. The V & D sulfides from garlic can reduce the LDL (low-density lipoprotein), triglycerides, and total cholesterol, and they can increase the HDL (high density lipoprotein). These V & D sulfides rebalance the fats in the blood back to a more normal level, thus reducing the risks of heart attacks and strokes.

It is interesting that the active V & D sulfides actually inactivate the enzyme that produces cholesterol in a much safer way than the cholesterol lowering drugs called statins. These V & D sulfides also block the effects of inflammatory chemicals produced by the white cells of the body. This is particularly important inside the arteries where the linings of the arteries are attacked by inflammatory chemicals. The garlic V & D sulfides are therefore protective against damage to the main blood vessels and reduce the likelihood of atherosclerosis progressing rapidly. Diabetics are particularly prone to artery disease and are protected by the garlic V & D sulfides.

The V & D sulfides also increase the activity of detoxifying enzymes. This is of great benefit to everybody, but it is of even greater benefit to a diabetic who may have high blood pressure, heart disease, and other health problems for which they may be taking medications. By activating the detoxifying enzymes, the V & D sulfides from the garlic will assist in removing the toxic byproducts of these medications.

Another advantage is that these compounds in garlic stimulate an increase in the production of heat by the body. This is done in the deep fatty tissues and may aid in weight control programs. The compounds in garlic also increase the metabolic rate, which means that the body burns up fuels at a faster rate. It is believed that the garlic compounds stimulate both the brain and the hormone glands to achieve this increased metabolic rate.

Garlic V & D sulfides also reduce blood sugar and improve glucose intolerance in diabetic animals. The sulfide used in these studies in rats performed better than both insulin and oral medications. These compounds in garlic are believed to increase the secretion of insulin from the pancreas and/or free the insulin in the blood to do its work.

Garlic V & D sulfides can act as antibiotics as they can kill both bacteria and fungi. The bug that causes stomach ulcers is called Helicobacter and garlic works against this bacterium.

The V & D sulfides also protect against oxidation damage and they reduce the activity of the sticky little platelets in the blood that cause clots to form. Garlic also reduces the ability of enzymes in the bloodstream to break down the fibrous material in blood clots. This means that if there is a tendency to produce blood clots that may result in a heart attack, stroke or kidney damage, the long-term use of garlic V & D sulfides may be protective against new clots forming.

In patients with the metabolic syndrome, there is a constellation of risk factors that can lead to the development of type 2 diabetes and cardiovascular disease. This may come about as a consequence of increased insulin resistance— that is, the cells of the body do not respond so well to the presence of insulin. As discussed earlier, metabolic syndrome is diagnosed in the presence of three of the following: abdominal obesity, high triglycerides, high levels of "bad" LDL cholesterol, high blood pressure, and high fasting blood glucose. (Refer to Chapter 1 for more detailed information about metabolic syndrome.) Of all of these conditions, fat loss in the abdominal area is the priority. If you can reduce your waist circumference and deep abdominal fat, all the other risk factors are reduced as well. There is also some very good evidence that the active components from garlic have a positive health effect on fat cells; that is, the garlic V & D sulfides make fat cells smaller. Fat cells in the abdominal region are very active. They produce the chemicals of inflammation, the chemicals stimulating appetite, and the chemicals that produce blood clots. These little fat cells are very actively destroying your body. They need to be starved out of existence. But they are very resistant to starvation.

The use of garlic V & D sulfides can play an extremely important role in assisting patients with prediabetes, diabetes and the metabolic syndrome to reduce the bad cholesterol, triglycerides and total cholesterol. This definitely works in favor of the person trying to lose weight and gain health.

PERMEABLE CURCUMIN FROM TURMERIC

Turmeric is a root vegetable commonly used in Indian curries. Turmeric gives curries their bright orange color and distinctive flavor. Most turmeric comes from India and there are many different varieties. Turmeric has been used in Indian medicine traditionally for many conditions, especially those associated with inflammation. Its traditional uses have been for rheumatic pains, arthritis, rheumatoid arthritis, poor vision, coughs and colds, and even for the stimulation of milk production. It is not uncommonly used for intestinal complaints. Therefore its wide use is an indication of its wide spectrum of activity.

The active component in turmeric is known as curcumin. Curcumin can act as an antioxidant and protect against oxidation damage to cells and tissues and it is a powerful anti-inflammatory agent. It also protects the liver and other tissues from the harmful effects of toxic chemicals. It may also reduce the stickiness of the blood platelets that cause clots. There are also some very good scientific studies and some animal studies to show that curcumin protects against cancer.

Turmeric is very safe and it has been used in Indian cooking for centuries. The amount of curcumin in turmeric is quite low, however, and may be only about 4% of the turmeric powder. Another of the major problems with using turmeric is that the curcumins are not very soluble in water. This means that it is very difficult to get the curcumin is at high concentration into areas of the body in which it is needed. With these low levels and with its low solubility, very large amounts of turmeric powder must be used to achieve a therapeutic effects.

A number of attempts to improve curcumin's solubility have been made, and a powerful form has been developed that can penetrate the cell membrane to perform its important functions within the cells of the body. Probably the best available curcumin is a substance called cumerone. Cumerone has been shown to pass through the cell membrane 11,000 times more effectively than ordinary curcumin. This makes it an extremely useful form of curcumin to be used in inflammatory conditions. It can be used instead of the non-steroid or anti-inflammatory drugs known as Cox two inhibitors for the treatment of muscular aches and pains, inflammation and arthritis. In fact it is quite fast acting and very safe. The only time that curcumin should not be used is if a patient has had an obstructed bile duct or active gallstones.

You may ask for the reason that I am mentioning turmeric and curcumin in a book on diabetes. There is good evidence that diabetics, pre-diabetics and people with the metabolic syndrome suffer from a low-grade to moderate grade inflammatory process in some of their organ systems. If there is associated severe overweight condition or obesity, there is no doubt that the breakdown of deep fat in the abdomen produces a chronic low-grade inflammation. The destruction of the pancreas also results in chronic low-grade inflammation. The wide variety of chemicals produced by fat cells in the gut and the harmful effects on the heart and blood vessels as well as the kidneys are inflammatory. The anti-inflammatory diet of fish or vegetables, fruits, nuts, berries, and seeds helps to prevent heart disease. diabetes, and many cancers. By simply adding turmeric with its curcumin to your treatment regime, I am ensuring that the anti-inflammatory diet (the Mediterranean diet) is augmented with one of nature's safest and most effective natural anti-inflammatory agents.

Scientific studies have proven that not only is curcumin and anti-inflammatory agent but it is also a powerful antioxidant, anti allergy, antispasmodic antibacterial, antifungal and anti-cancer substance. When the medical and scientific community catch up with a better understanding of the process by which foods and chemicals can cause inflammation, the use of a fast acting anti-inflammatory such as curcumin in the long-term management of patients with diabetes will become appreciated and used as a part of mainstream healthcare. The other aspect of curcumin is that if it can penetrate the cell and nuclear membranes, it has the ability to alter the expression of many genes. As an anti-inflammatory agent it acts on the genes.

The daily use of turmeric or a highly bioavailable curcumin will help maintain the best of health for people with or without diabetes.

CINNAMON

Cinnamon is a well-known spice that is used in cooking savory and sweet foods. It is obtained from the inside of the bark of the cinnamon tree that is native to India and Asia. Cinnamon has a characteristic taste and smell and is one of the most pleasant spices to use.

As a spice used for medicinal purposes, cinnamon has been used for the common cold, as well as the relief of diarrhea and abdominal pains of unknown cause. It is a powerful antioxidant and the essential oil of cinnamon has antibacterial and possibly antiviral properties as well. It can aid in the preservation of foods and drinks. More recently scientific and clinical studies have shown that cinnamon may be effective in the treatment of type 2 diabetes, insulin resistance, and metabolic syndrome. The cinnamon that has been used for the study of diabetes is from the Chinese cinnamon tree and the active ingredient is called cinnamon tanning B_1. Other actions of extracts of cinnamon include the possible prevention of cancer of the bowel and malignant melanoma.

Animal studies have shown that whole cinnamon and aqueous or water extracts of cinnamon can reduce blood pressure elevations caused by high sugar intake in rats. A diet high in sugar causes insulin resistance and high blood pressure. There are now a number of human studies that confirm cinnamon and cinnamon extracts are useful in reducing fasting blood sugar levels in people with type 2 diabetes, reducing blood sugar levels after a meal, slowing the emptying of food from the stomach, reducing glycated hemoglobin (HbA1C), and improving insulin sensitivity. Doses of cinnamon of 1 to 3 g per day are effective.

In many of these studies the subjects have been healthy individuals and the use of cinnamon in type 2 diabetes can be recommended. The dose required is in the range of 3 to 6 g per day. However, a German study has recommended that those with poor blood sugar control may benefit from supplementation with cinnamon using a high-quality cinnamon powder, tablet or capsule. The long-term use of cinnamon in type 2 diabetes to maintain a low level of HbA1C is of great advantage in the prevention of complications. There is no good reason for denying a patient with type 1 diabetes the use of this valuable spice. Also, the combined use of different herbs and spices in the management of the patient with diabetes is probably better than using a high potent dose of any single spice. Most of these plant materials are very gentle in nature, very safe even for long-term use and extremely forgiving in the case of an overdose. Remember, it is wise to take the recommended doses of the manufacturer or your healthcare practitioner.

GYMNEMA SYLVESTRE

Gymnema is a native herb that inhabits the tropical rainforests of India. It has been used as an herbal medicine for the treatment of diabetes for almost 2,000 years. Gymnema contains organic acids that have an anti-inflammatory action, and an anti-diabetic activity. One of the most important actions of gymnema is that it can stimulate the secretion of insulin from the pancreas. To achieve this it requires an adequate amount of calcium. The leaves of the plant have been used to reduce blood sugar levels. The herb is very gentle and it reduces the blood sugar slowly over a long period of time. Gymnema has also been shown to have an anti-sweetness action; it reduces the taste of sugar and so can be used for reducing the cravings for sweets and sugar rich foods. It works in a slightly different way to reducing sugar cravings compared to the minerals chromium and zinc. In addition to reducing the desire for sweets, gymnema also reduces the transport of sugars across the intestine. It also reduces the transport of fatty acids across the intestine and into the blood. Therefore, gymnema has a number of actions very beneficial to the health of people with diabetes.

The use of Gymnema in diabetes must be considered in conjunction with all the other available natural health products and the selection of which to use is often best left to a properly trained professional.

PANAX GINSENG

In a study involving 19 participants with well-controlled type 2 diabetes adhering to their usual anti-diabetic therapy (diet and/or medications), supplementation with panax ginseng was found to improve glucose and insulin regulation. The participants were to receive either a placebo or a selected Korean red ginseng preparation (2 g/meal = 6 g/day; taken orally, 40 minutes before meal) for a period of 12 weeks.

Panax ginseng supplementation led to no change in HbA1c, but this may have been due to the short duration of the study. However, the participants remained well controlled (HbA1c = 6.5%) throughout the treatment period. Additionally, panax ginseng supplementation was found to decrease blood glucose after a sugar challenge by 8–11%, decrease fasting plasma insulin by 33–38%, and increase fasting insulin sensitivity by 33%, compared to placebo.

The authors of this study conclude that "Although clinical efficacy, as assessed by HbA1c, was not demonstrated, 12 weeks of supplementation with the selected ginseng treatment maintained good sugar control and improved blood glucose and blood insulin regulation safely beyond usual therapy in people with well-controlled type 2 diabetes."

American ginseng, a different species to the Panax, reduces high blood glucose levels in type 2 diabetics and non-diabetics. If American ginseng is given to non-diabetics, it should be given with meals to prevent hypoglycemia.

Ginseng is of great value during periods of stress. It is also known as an adaptogenic herb—something that helps you to adapt and cope with stressful situations.

TAURINE

Taurine is a sulfur-containing amino acid that is found in fish and meat. Unfortunately, the flavor-enhancing substance MSG destroys taurine, mercury reduces its absorption, and both chemotherapy and radiotherapy cause depletion.

Selenium is found in very high concentrations in the muscle of the heart. Taurine helps the trace element selenium to move into cells. Taurine is found in the bile secreted by the gallbladder and helps digestion. It also prevents the formation of gallstones. It stabilizes the cell membranes of the brain and the heart. It binds on to heavy metals such as aluminum and arsenic and helps to excrete them from the body. Like selenium, taurine also supports the immune system.

Taurine is important in people with diabetes because it helps to normalize the amount of potassium in heart muscle cells. Potassium is an important mineral in diabetics and needs to be carefully balanced. If a diabetic also has coronary artery disease and is at risk of a heart attack, the presence of taurine at optimal levels in the heart will reduce serious disturbances in heart rhythm after a heart attack, thus reducing the likelihood of a fatality. Taurine makes the electrical activity in the heart and its rhythm normal. Diabetics who suffer from congestive heart failure also benefit from taurine supplementation. Taurine also prevents abnormal blood clotting, it lowers cholesterol and it lowers blood pressure. High doses of taurine, for example 6 g per day, over a week, can reduce blood pressure. Taurine can also act as a fluid tablet (a diuretic) without the side effects of diuretic drugs that push out trace elements in the urine. It may also be beneficial in the diabetic with nephropathy (kidney disease).

Taurine is important in the health of the eye. It accumulates in the retina and a deficiency of taurine will result in the degeneration of the retina. Supplementation with taurine helps to prevent and may reverse macular degeneration. In these situations it should never be considered by itself. Always remember, nutrients work in groups.

Taurine works with insulin receptors to improve their function. It may be low in insulin-dependent diabetics. Supplementation with taurine definitely improves the action of insulin. It also reduces the stickiness of the blood platelets and it protects against the damaging effects of diabetes on the lining of blood vessels. It may also be useful in cases of male infertility where there is sperm with poor mobility. Taurine also enhances the production of bile salts thus improving digestion especially in the diabetic who has liver disease. Because of its ability to stabilize the nervous system, taurine may also be useful in the diabetic with liver disease who is having difficulty coming off alcohol. It also speeds up the breakdown of alcohol.

SAME: S-ADENOSYL METHIONINE

SAMe is another sulfur containing amino acid. It is important in helping to maintain a normal healthy mood, nerve function, brain function, and intellect. It can also help to reduce tiredness and morning stiffness, and it can improve the health of the liver.

SAMe is known as a methyl donor; it is involved in the manufacture of a wide range of important biochemicals in the body. It is essential for the formation of the chemicals in the brain and in the manufacture of many other cell chemicals including proteins, lipids, DNA and RNA. Healthy liver detoxification cannot occur without SAMe.

Heart and blood vessel diseases are common in diabetics. One of the chemicals produced by the body that causes heart disease is homocysteine. SAMe assists in the removal of homocysteine. SAMe also helps in the production of glutathione, another important antioxidant that has recently been found to be deficient in the brains of patients with severe depression, schizophrenia, bipolar disorder and autism spectrum disorder. In diabetes, one of the most common symptoms is depression. A change in diet, exercise and a choice of appropriate supplement can do wonders compared to drugs in these situations. Glutathione levels in the brain can be improved with injections of glutathione, sublingual glutathione tablets, SAMe or another amino acid called NAC. These supplements can produce improvements in all of these conditions, although SAMe should not be given to someone with mania.

SAMe is very safe and has very few side-effects. It may cause mild nausea or constipation in some patients. If it is given with vitamin B complex, the mild restlessness that occasionally occurs from SAMe is easily controlled. SAMe should not be given to patients with a history of mania unless they are closely monitored.

PROBIOTICS

Apart from a change to a vegetarian style of diet and the use of nutritional supplements and herbs, one of the most efficient ways of improving the health of the intestines and their contents is the use of probiotic supplements. These are the friendly bacteria including Lactobacillus and Bifidobacteria. Probiotics need to be selected very carefully and should be recommended by a qualified healthcare practitioner. There are many probiotics on the market that claim to have superior effect because of clinical studies that have been performed on them. However many of these clinical studies have been funded by the companies that make the probiotics. It is probably best to avoid probiotics that are commercially promoted on the basis of clinical studies funded by the parent company. Healthcare practitioners with experience in the use of probiotics can provide the best advice. The advice I can give you here is that if you suffer from either type 1 or type 2 diabetes, the use of a probiotic powder or capsule with each meal will ensure that gut health can be optimized very easily with this approach. Try to avoid probiotic tablets as the bacteria become less stable from the heat of the tableting process. There are also probiotics on the market that do not undergo proper stability studies. This means that you cannot be sure that the number of live bacteria in the capsule is correct. In fact I have had probiotics tested in which there are no live bacteria remaining. Every batch of probiotic needs to be tested.

In addition to the above recommendations, another very good treatment is the use of a raw food diet, either intermittently or continuously.

RAW FOODS AND UNPROCESSED FOODS

There is a lot of good anecdotal evidence that the use of raw foods, that is, foods that have not been cooked, may be useful for weight reduction. Raw foods still contain active enzymes that assist in the digestion and assimilation of the nutrients contained in the foods. In addition raw foods contain more of the nutrients that are often destroyed by the heating and cooking process. This is not to say that cooked foods are not healthy because with

AND DON'T FORGET EXERCISE

Did you know that adding a walk to the daily routine not only helps you shed pounds but it also powerfully boosts your insulin sensitivity? The further you walk the greater the benefits.

Recent studies in Australia have shown that if you increase your daily step count over five years, you will have a lower Body Mass Index, smaller waist-to-hip ratio and higher insulin sensitivity than if you remain sedentary.

Adults who go from relative inactivity to walking 10,000 steps per day can expect to boost their insulin sensitivity three times, compared with an inactive person who took up walking 3,000 steps per day. This is absolutely wonderful news for those of us who like gentle exercise and just cannot bear the thought of pounding the pavements or even working up a mild sweat.

Increasing the daily step count to 10,000 (about 5 miles) over 5 years significantly reduces your Body Mass Index. This is a long, slow but sure process that I would find hard to believe anyone who can walk objecting to.

cooking some nutrients are made more available to the body. So it's important here to find the right balance. I would suggest that if you are interested in the raw food diet, there are a number of experts available who can assist to ensure that the diet is balanced and you get all the nutrients you require. Nude foods are foods that are not dressed up with commercially available sauces, dressings and other condiments. You don't know what you are eating if you are consuming these pre-prepared substances that come out of bottles and cans. If you are going to use dressings, ensure that the raw ingredients are as pure as possible and free of chemical contaminants such as colorings, flavorings, preservatives and emulsifiers etc. Importantly, avoid the polyunsaturated oils from sunflower and safflower and use cold pressed virgin olive oil.

The research confirms that walking 10,000 steps per day can ward off diabetes in the average person. The benefits of walking are independent of dietary energy intake and the effect of walking was largely due to a reduction in fatness (adiposity).

And the other benefits are that walking like this helps people with both type1 and type 2 diabetes, those with anxiety and depression and even those who are afraid of exercise. It's a nice habit to get into. Walking like this is an effective and powerful form of meditation without the crap. Don't forget to breathe in through your nose to produce all those healthy benefits of nasal breathing including the healthy happy biochemicals made in the nose when the air flows past (scientifically proven).

Remember that exercise is stressful and a little stress is good. Don't overdo it to the point where you get tired, sore muscles and shortness of breath. Feel good at the end of an exercise session. Don't forget that your antioxidant diet and supplements will give you the energy to do more exercise safely and protect you against the oxidating free radicals generated by the exercise.

Dark green leafy vegetables contain significant amounts of chlorophyll, the green pigment found in leafy vegetables. Chlorophyll is a very powerful detoxifying agent and it assists in maintaining the healthy bacteria in the gut. It also assists in reducing and neutralizing the toxins produced by some of the bad bacteria. It is also a very rich source of magnesium, which is very important in the diabetic but it is also useful in ensuring that healthy bowel actions are formed every day, preferably more than once. This is all part of the detoxification process. You will notice how much better you feel.

CHAPTER 11

SUPPLEMENTS FOR DIABETICS

*Of several remedies, the physician should
choose the least sensational.*
—HIPPOCRATES

In my opinion, nutritional supplements should be recommended
for all diabetics. *There is not a single diabetic who will not benefit from appropriate and judicial supplementation.* To correct
imbalances and deficiencies that contribute to suboptimal diabetic and metabolic control, and to prevent diabetic complications, should be the aim of every physician. It is medical
negligence to ignore the scientific literature on the health benefits of supplementation in prediabetes, types 1 and 2 diabetes,
gestational diabetes, metabolic syndrome and those with a
genetic predisposition to diabetes. Attempts to correct deficiencies and imbalances with diet alone is, at best unscientific, and
at worst, gross medical negligence. It is about time that doctors
were properly trained in nutritional medicine before they are ever
unleashed onto the public.

This does not mean that orthodox medicine should be ignored,
but in diabetes, it should be relegated to second place in every
instance except for the severe diabetic and those with an urgent
need for intensive hospital care, such as diabetic ketoacidosis,
coma, or other emergency.

RECOMMENDED SUPPLEMENTS

Caution: The doses below are doses commonly administered by nutritional (orthomolecular) practitioners. They should not be casually self-prescribed by patients. Individuals who may wish to use these supplements should do so with due care, including the observation and adherence to the doses recommended on the label, and the avoidance of supplements causing drug interactions

GOALS OF NUTRITIONAL SUPPLEMENTATION FOR PERSONS WITH DIABETES

- protect the pancreas and other organs from the damaging effects of free radicals

- increase the likelihood of the pancreas to make, store, and release more insulin

- enhance the activity of the insulin available to the body's cells

- increase levels of antioxidants to slow the aging process and retard progression of diseases and their complications

- support and stimulate the immune system to fight infection and reduce the damage caused by any autoimmune process

- reduce the risks of cancer, heart disease, stroke, kidney disease, eye disease, osteoporosis, gangrene and killer infections

- reduce cholesterol and triglycerides

- improve wound healing

- increase mental and physical well-being enabling effective exercise to be performed

- provide important anti-inflammatory and pro-healing nutrients to allow the resolution of chronic inflammation in the deep fat of the gut

if the person is taking medication. Your own nutritional program needs to first be discussed with, and then monitored by, your personal physician.

VITAMINS

Vitamin C containing a mixture of the different forms of vitamin C and a mixture of bioflavonoids including quercetin. The dose ranges from 1,000–8,000 mg/day. Take as powder, capsules, or tablets.

Vitamin E Complex containing a mixture of the tocopherols and tocotrienols: 500–1,000 IU/day

High Potency Vitamin B-Complex containing a balance of the B vitamins for maximum efficacy.

Niacinamide (Vitamin B$_3$): 500–2,000 mg/day

Pyridoxine (Vitamin B$_6$): 100–300 mg/day

Folic Acid: 0.5–1 mg/day

Methylcobalamin (special vitamin B$_{12}$): 1,000 or more micrograms/day

Vitamin D: 1,000–5,000 units/day

MINERALS AND TRACE ELEMENTS

Magnesium as Orotate, Chelate or Aspartate: 200–600 mg/day

Zinc as Chelate, Picolinate or Methionate: 30—60 mg/day

Chromium as Chelate or Picolinate: 500–2,000 mcg/day

Vanadium as Vanadyl sulfate: 30 mg/day

Selenium as selenomethionine: 200–400 mcg/day

OTHER NUTRIENTS

Fish Oil Omega-3: 3 g/day

Primrose Oil Omega-6: 1 g/day

Inositol: 3–6 g/day

Alpha Lipoic Acid: 500–1,000 mg/day

Acetyl L-Carnitine: 1,000–6,000 mg/day

Taurine: 400–800 mg/day

VEGETABLE JUICES

Carrot and beetroot: to supply carotenoids as natural broad-spectrum antioxidants for heart, kidney, brain and eye health and protection

May I offer a word to the wise? Self-discipline is less hampering than chronic ill-health.

AFTERWORD

It never ceases to amaze me how many beneficial actions nutrients have and how few side effects, if any, there are. Compare this to drugs, which usually have a single action and lists of adverse reactions, some lethal. I am a medical doctor. The statement I just made is not typical of medical doctors. I would like to tell you about myself so that you, the reader of this book, may have a better understanding of the reasons that I have chosen a different path: the practice of nutritional and natural medicine.

Before I studied medicine, I first had earned a degree in Agricultural Science in 1965. For the following three years I was involved in teaching and research. My research interests were in the fields of agricultural science and animal nutrition, including the nutritional health of cattle, horses, sheep, dogs, pigs and poultry. I was also intensely interested in fruit and vegetable production, soil science, and the use and misuse of herbicides and pesticides in food production. I was formulating foods including the addition of micronutrients (vitamins and trace minerals) to improve the fertility, growth rates, performance and productivity of animals.

However, I was extremely disillusioned by the way food for people was being produced, even way back in the 1960s. The proposals by the food industry regarding mass production of more and ever-more highly processed foods containing multitudes of additives shocked me. My grandfather was a brilliant chef. In the early twentieth century, he had cooked in many of the most famous locations in Europe. He always emphasized fresh, whole, clean food be used in the preparation of a meal that we sat down to eat, and always together. No cans or packets of food in his house. He actually introduced olive oil and garlic into some of Australia's top hotels. My grandparents died in their sleep in their late 80s without a day of serious illness.

I became interested in health, had some friends in the medical profession, and decided to do a medical course. In 1969 I entered medical school at the University of New South Wales and completed my clinical studies at Monash University in Victoria, graduating as a physician and surgeon in 1974. I enjoyed the first three years of the course because it was about science; it was during the clinical years that I became concerned about my training to become a doctor.

Patient after patient I was seeing as a medical student were receiving what I was told was the best medical care in the world. Many of them were not really getting any healthier and their illnesses were progressing. The difference between my agricultural science training and my medical training was that nutritional sciences were brought into nearly every aspect of agriculture, from the nutrients in the soil, to the orchard, horticulture, breeding of sheep, production of meat in cattle, productivity of dairy cows, growth rates of pigs. We had only four hours of "nutrition" in a six year medical course. It doesn't make a lot of sense to know so little about a topic when it's going to be the reason that over ninety percent of your patients are going to die.

A little old lady lying in bed after major surgery for cancer is not regarded as a productive animal. That is unfortunate for her. She receives intravenous sugar, salt and water, is fed overcooked everything, and eats meals including sweets such as ice cream and gelatin desserts. Not a vitamin bottle in sight.

She is obviously malnourished. She is a very interesting "case" for the professor of medicine and his students. One student requests some information about the lady's diet and nutritional status. The professor retorts that "this lady's diet has nothing to do with her current state; now we'll move on to her real problems." By the way, that student was me. That professor's response disgusted me and that was the turning point in my profession. I reflect on the ignorance in my profession, and when I do, I am reminded of that particular professor. I am also reminded about the wonderful training doctors get and how clever they are, that cleverness being matched and in some cases exceeded by their ignorance and arrogance believing that pharmaceutical and surgical medicine is the only true and scientific route to health.

After completing my residency and a year of general medicine and anesthetic practice, I traveled widely throughout Europe, North America and Asia searching for solutions to the problems created by the significant gaps that I had recognized in the normal medical training of doctors. This educational travel included a six month appointment as a ship surgeon, with travel to many parts of the world. This travel and educational process to learn about all forms of medicine and healing has continued throughout my nearly 40 years of practice as a doctor. I specialized in nutritional and environmental medicine with particular interests in cancer, psychiatric illness, auto-immune diseases, diabetes, learning and behavioral disorders, heart disease, psychological disorders related to foods and chemicals, the chronic fatigue syndrome, arthritis, asthma, and food and chemical sensitivities.

For decades, I have been closely involved in the establishment of Integrative Medicine. The intravenous vitamin C clinics that I developed were the first of their kind in Australia. Then, in the early 1980s, I had another life-changing event. A very sick man heard about my intravenous vitamin C clinic. He visited and asked me to treat him. He had full-blown AIDS including the Kaposis' Sarcoma cancer. At the time I saw him, the stage of his disease offered him a life expectancy of a mere 11 months; a very poor prognosis. I will call him Jack.

Jack routinely visited the clinic for treatments which, for the time being were megadoses of intravenous vitamin C, the doses I was successfully using in my cancer and leukemia patients, and mistletoe injections, to stimulate healthy white cells. He discovered that with this treatment he stopped growing new Kaposis cancers, which are dark blue to black lumps on the skin including the face; some of his existing Kaposis had disappeared.

Jack's 11 month prognosis was incorrect. He lived for another 9 years, dying eventually from AIDS-Related Dementia. Nine years beats 11 months any way you look at it. Thus motivated, I wrote and published a book called "The AIDS Fighters" (Keats Publishing, 1986).

My activities, and this book, provoked some medical professionals to complain to the Medical Board about my using nutrients and high doses of intravenous vitamin C to treat cancer and HIV/AIDS patients. The medical board had decided to hold an enquiry. If I was found guilty of any single charge, they would strike me off and I would never be able to practice medicine again. For someone who came from a background unfamiliar with the medico-legal establishment, this came as a shock; an even bigger shock when there were over 16 charges of "infamous conduct in a professional respect." Infamous conduct in a professional respect is the sort of charge the Medical Board reserves for doctors who commit heinous crimes against their patients. None of my patients were harmed, and most lived longer and healthier lives from the type of treatments they received.

I didn't come from a wealthy family; I won a scholarship to medical school and now saw that all my efforts would be in vain if I lost my license to practice. The hearing lasted for four days under a now-reduced charge of professional misconduct (mind you, for publishing scientifically-based works that didn't appeal to some in the medical profession). I was found guilty, reprimanded, and fined $5,000, a lot of money those days. I appealed to the Supreme Court and won. The medical board was severely criticized by the Court and was ordered to pay my costs.

Since that case, I have been active in helping other doctors fight the injustices dealt to them by a medical system and its allied institutions, including government, that have improved very little since then, despite the consumer's preference for more natural health care. I also pioneered the first post-graduate medical course in nutrition in Australia, remaining on the faculty for 27 years.

The attacks by medical boards, the AMA, and government on doctors who prefer vitamins over drugs are truly abhorrent to me. I continue to lobby politicians for change to a more sustainable health system. Please join me in this effort. Write to your elected representatives, medical societies, insurance companies, hospitals, and newspapers and tell them that you want unfettered, unrestricted access to high-dose nutritional therapy, intravenous vitamin C, and other natural health care modalities.

BIBLIOGRAPHY

SUGAR AND DIABETES

"Eat Less Sugar," *The Lancet,* December 23/30 1989; 1538.

American Diabetes Association. Clinical Practice Recommendations 1998. "Position Statement: Nutrition recommendations and principles for people with diabetes mellitus." *Diabetes Care,* 1998; 21(Suppl 1).

Apovian, C.M., "Sugar-Sweetened Soft Drinks, Obesity, and Type 2 Diabetes," *JAMA,* August 25, 2004; 292(8):978–979.

Brand-Miller, Janette C., "Importance of glycemic index in diabetes," *American Journal of Clinical Nutrition,* 1994; 59(Suppl.):747S–752S.

Cohen, A.M., et al., "Experimental models in diabetes." *Sugars in Nutrition.* San Francisco, Academic Press, 1974; 483–511.

Frayn, K.N., Kingman, S.M., "Dietary sugars and lipid metabolism in humans." *Am J Clin Nutr,* 1995; 62(Suppl):250S–63S.

Gabel, Lawrence, Ph.D., et al., "Dietary prevention and treatment of disease," *AFP Journal,* November 1992; 415–485.

Hallfrisch, J., et al., "Effects of dietary fructose on plasma glucose and hormone responses in normal and hyperinsulinemic man." *J Nutr,* 1983; 113:1819–26.

Kozlovsky, A.S., et al., "Effects of diets high in simple sugars on urinary chromium losses." *Metabolism,* 1986; 35(6):515–18.

Malerbi, D.A., et al., "Metabolic effects of dietary sucrose and fructose in type II diabetic subjects." *Diabetes Care,* 1996; 19(11):1249–56.

Mayer-Davis, E.J., et al., "Dietary fat and insulin sensitivity in a triethnic population: the role of obesity." The Insulin Resistance Atherosclerosis Study (IRAS). *Am J Clin Nutr,* 1997; 65:79–87.

"Mellitus in women." *JAMA,* 1997; 277(6):472–7.

Parillo, M., et al., "Does a high carbohydrate diet have different effects in NIDDM patients treated with diet alone or hypoglycemic drugs?" *Diabetes Care,* 1996; 19(5):498–500.

Reiser, S., et al., "Blood lipids, lipoproteins, apoproteins, and uric acid in men fed diets containing fructose or high-amylose cornstarch." *Am J Clin Nutr,* 1989; 49:832–9.

Reiser, S., et al., "Effects of sugars on indices of glucose tolerance in humans." *Am J Clin Nutr,* 1986; 43(1):151–9.

Ruhe, R.C., McDonald, R.B., "Use of antioxidant nutrients in the prevention and treatment of type 2 diabetes." *J Am Coll Nutr,* 2001; 20(suppl 5):363S–369S.

Salmeron, J., et al., "Dietary fiber, glycemic load, and risk of non-insulin-dependent diabetes."

Singh, R., Barden, A., Mori, T., Beilin, L., "Advanced glycation end-products: a review." *Diabetologia,* 2001; 44:129–46.

Storlien, L.H., et al., "Effects of sucrose vs starch diets on in vivo insulin action, thermogenesis, and obesity in rats." *Am J Clin Nutr,* 1988; 47:420–7.

Swade, T.F., Emanuele, N.V., "Alcohol & Diabetes." *Compr Ther,* 1997; 23(2):135–40.

Tanasescu, M., Hu, F.B., Willett, W.C., et al, "Alcohol consumption and risk of coronary heart disease among men with type 2 diabetes mellitus." *J Am Coll Cardiol,* 2001; 38:1836–42.

The Clinical Advisor, "Soft drinks implicated in type 2 diabetes." October 2004; 13.

Thorburn, A.W., et al., "Fructose-induced in vivo insulin resistance and elevated plasma triglyceride levels in rats." *Am J Clin Nutr,* 1989; 49:1155–63.

Virtanen, S.M., et al., "Is children's or parents' coffee or tea consumption associated with the risk for insulin-dependent diabetes mellitus in children?" *Eur J Clin Nutr,* 1994; 48:279–85.

Werbach, M.R., *Textbook of Nutritional Medicine,* Tarzana, CA, Third Line Press, 1999.

West, K.M., Kalbfleisch, J.M., "Influence of nutritional factors on prevalence of diabetes." *Diabetes,* 1971; 20:99–108.

Wise, Joyce, M.D., "Effect of sucrose-containing snacks on blood glucose control." *Diabetes Care,* June 1989; 12(6):423–426.

Yudkin, John, M.A., M.D., Ph.D., "Sugar and the diseases of affluence." *The Nutrition Report,* August 1989; 7(8):57–64.

Yudkin, John, M.D., "Report on The COMA panel on dietary sugars in human disease: Discussion paper." *Journal of The Royal Society of Medicine,* October 1990; 83:627–628.

FOOD ALLERGIES AND DIABETES

"Group blasts milk, ignites 'Food Terrorism' debate." *Nutrition Week,* October 9, 1992; 22(38):2.

Anderson, J.W., Quella, S.K., Yetley, E.A., "Sorting out health claims about soy." *Patient Care,* December 15, 2000; 14–28.

Atkinson, M.A., Ellis, T.M., "Infants diets and insulin-dependent diabetes: evaluating the "cows' milk hypothesis" and a role for anti-bovine serum albumin immunity." *J Am Coll Nutr,* 1997; 16(4):334–40.

Finberg, Laurence, M.D., "How good a food for humans is cow's milk? From Hyperbole Up to Hyperbole Down," *The American Journal of Diseases in Children,* December 1992; 146:1432.

Freed, D.L.J., "Do dietary lectins cause disease? The evidence is suggestive—and raises interesting possibilities for treatment." *BMJ,* April 17, 1999; 318:1023–1024.

Hedges, Harold H., M.D., "The elimination diet as a diagnostic tool." *AFP Journal,* November 1992; 46(5):77S–85S.

Kang, J.H., Tsuyoshi, G., et al., "Dietary capsaicin reduces obesity-induced insulin resistance and hepatic steatosis in obese mice fed a high-fat diet." *Obesity,* 2009

Kitts, David, et al., "Adverse reactions to food constituents: allergy, intolerance, and autoimmunity." *Canadian Journal of Physiology and Pharmacology,* 1997; 75:241–254.

Kohno, T., Kobashiri, Y., Sugie, Y., et al., "Antibodies to food antigens in Japanese patients with type 1 diabetes mellitus." *Diabetes Res Clin Pract,* 2002; 55:1–9.

Kostraba, J.N., et al., "Nitrate levels in community drinking waters and risk of IDDM. An ecological analysis." *Diabetes Care,* 1992; 15(11):1505–8.

Murphy, Neil, J., M.D., et al., "Dietary change and obesity associated with glucose intolerance in Alaska natives." *Journal of the American Dietetic Association,* June 1995; 95 (6):676–681.

Murray, R., Frankowski, B., et al., "Are soft drinks a scapegoat for childhood obesity?" *J Pediatr,* May 2005; 146:586–590.

Neyestani, T.R., Shariat-Zadeh, N., et al., "The opposite associations of lycopene and body fat mass with humoral immunity in type 2 diabetes mellitus: a possible role in atherogenesis." *Iran J Allergy Asthma Immunol,* 2007; 6(2): 79–87.

Nikolaidis, L.A., Kounis, N.G., Gradman, A.H., "Allergic angina and allergic myocardial infarction: A new twist on an old syndrome." *Can J Cardiol,* May 2002; 18(5):508–511.

Pereira, M.A., Kartashov, A.I., et al., "Fast-food habits, weight gain, and insulin resistance (The CARDIA Study): 15-year prospective analysis." *Lancet,* January 1, 2005; 365:36–42.

Pereira, M.A., Liu, S., "Types of carbohydrates and risk of cardiovascular disease." *J Women's Health,* 2003; 12(2):115–122.

Power, R.A., Hulver, M.W., et al., "Carnitine revisited: potential use as adjunctive treatment in diabetes." *Diabetologia,* 2007; 50(4): 824–832.

Rabinowich, I.M., "Achlorhydria and its clinical significance in diabetes mellitus." *Am J Dig Dis,* 1949; 16:322–32.

Richardson, C.T., et al., "Diabetics have reduced acid secretion and delayed digestion. *Am Family Physician* June, 1978, p. 143

Scott FW et al. Milk and type 1 diabetes, Examining the evidence and broadening the focus." *Diabetes Care* 1996; 19(4):379–83.

Sheard, N.F., "The diabetic diet: evidence for a new approach." *Nutr Rev,* 1995; 53(1):16–18.

THE GENES OF DIABETES AND THE METABOLIC SYNDROME

American Diabetes Association, 2011.

Henry Erlich, Ana Maria Valdes, Janelle Noble, Joyce A. Carlson, Mike Varney, Pat Concannon, Josyf C. Mychaleckyj, John A. Todd, Persia Bonella, Anna Lisa Fear, Eva Lavant, Anthony Louey, Priscilla Moonsamy, for the Type 1 Diabetes Genetics Consortium "HLA DR-DQ Haplotypes and Genotypes and Type 1 Diabetes Risk Analysis of the Type 1 Diabetes Genetics Consortium Families" *Diabetes,* Vol 57, April 2008.

Park, Y., "Why is type 1 diabetes uncommon in Asia?" *Ann N Y Acad Sci,* Oct 2006; 1079:31–40.

Ridderstråle, M., Parikh, H., Groop. L., "Calpain 10 and type 2 diabetes: are we getting closer to an explanation?" *Curr Opin Clin Nutr Metab Care*, Jul 2005; 8(4):361–6.

Sadauskaite-Kuehne, V., et al., "Longer breastfeeding is an independent protective factor against development of type 1 diabetes mellitus in childhood." *Diabetes Metab Res Rev*, Mar-Apr 2004; 20(2):150–7.

PREDIABETES

Anderson, J.W., "Recent advances in carbohydrate nutrition and metabolism in diabetes mellitus." *J Am Coll Nutr*, 1989; 8(Suppl):61S–67S.

Chatfield, K., "Preventive medicine clinics: A case of diabetes." *Townsend Letter for Doctors*, March 1985; p. 105.

Colditz, G.A., et al., "Diet and risk of clinical diabetes in women." *Am J Clin Nutr*, 1992; 55:1018–23.

Dahlquist, G.G.. et al., "Dietary factors and the risk of developing insulin dependent diabetes in children.: *Br Med J*, 1990; 300:1302–6.

Heine, R.J., et al., "Linoleic-acid-enriched diet: Long-term effects on serum lipoprotein and apolipoprotein concentrations and insulin sensitivity in noninsulin-dependent diabetic patients." *Am J Clin Nutr*, 1989; 49:448–56.

Henriksen, E.J., "Exercise training and the antioxidant alpha-lipoic acid in the treatment of insulin resistance and type 2 diabetes." *Free Radic Biol Med*, 2006; 40(1): 3–12.

Kwak, J.H., Chae, J.S., et al., "Black soy - Peptide supplementation improves glucose control in subjects with prediabetes and newly diagnosed type 2 diabetes mellitus." *J Med Food*, 2010; 13(6): 1307–12.

Maddox, R., Maddox, S., "Choosing wellness: prevention of type 2 diabetes." *U.S. Pharmacist*, November 2004; 66–70.

National Institutes of Health Consensus Development Conference (USA), December 1986.

SOFT DRINKS AND CHILDHOOD OBESITY

Mrdjenovic and Levitsky, *J Pediatr*, 2003; 142:604–610.

Schwartz in *J Pediatr*, 2003; 142:599–601.

TYPE 1 DIABETES

Buyken, A.E., Toeller, M., Heitkamp, G., et al., "Eurodiab IDDM Complications Study Group. Glycemic index in the diet of European outpatients with type 1 diabetes: relations to glycated hemoglobin and serum lipids." *Am J Clin Nutr*, 2001;73:574–81.

Buyken, A.E., Toeller, M., Heitkamp, G., et al., "Glycemic index in the diet of European outpatients with type 1 diabetes: relations to glycated hemoglobin and serum lipids." *Am J Clin Nutr*, 2001; 73:574–81.

Christiansen, E., et al., "Intake of a diet high in *trans* monounsaturated fatty acids or saturated fatty acids. Effects on postprandial insulinemia and glycemia in obese patients with NIDDM." *Diabetes Care*, 1997; 20(5):881–7.

Fish, L.H., "Diabetic ketoacidosis. Treatment strategies to avoid complications.: *Postgrad Med*, 1994; 96(3):75–8.

Hollenbeck, C.B., et al., "The composition and nutritional adequacy of subject-selected high carbohydrate, low fat diets in insulin-dependent diabetes mellitus." *Am J Clin Nutr,* 1983; 38(1):41–51.

Osterode, W., et al., "Nutritional antioxidants, red cell membrane fluidity and blood viscosity in type I (insulin dependent) diabetes mellitus." *Diabetic Med,* 1996; 13:1044–50.

Schmetterer, L., et al., "Nitric oxide and ocular blood flow in patients with IDDM." *Diabetes,* 1997; 46(4):653–8.

Tong, H.I., "Influence of neurotropic vitamins on the nerve conduction velocity in diabetic neuropathy." *Ann Acad Med Singapore,* 1980; 9(1):65–70.

NUTRIENTS FOR THE TREATMENT OF DIABETES—MOVING TO A CURE

Anderson, R.A., Roussel, A.M., Zouari, N., et al., "Potential antioxidant effects of zinc and chromium supplementation in people with type 2 diabetes mellitus." *J Am Coll Nutr,* 2001; 20–212–8.

Chen, M.D., et al., "Selected metals status in patients with noninsulin-dependent diabetes mellitus." *Biol Trace Elem Res,* 1995; 50:119–24.

Crane, M.G., Sample, C., "Regression of diabetic neuropathy with total vegetarian (vegan) diet." *J Nutr Med,* 1994; 4:431–9.

Crary, E.J., McCarty, M.F., "Potential clinical applications for high-dose nutritional antioxidants." *Med Hypotheses,* 1984; 13:77–98.

Cunningham, J.J., "Altered vitamin C transport in diabetes mellitus." *Med Hypotheses,* 1988; 26:263–5.

Freyler, H., "Modern trends in the treatment of diabetic retinopathy." *Wien Klin Wochenschr,* 1977; 89(4):101–6.

Hughes, T.A., et al., "Glycemic responses in insulin-dependent diabetic patients: effect of food composition." *Am J Clin Nutr,* 1989; 49:658–66.

Kahler, W., et al., "Diabetes mellitus: a free radical-associated disease. Results of adjuvant antioxidant supplementation." *Z Gesamte Inn Med,* 1993; 48(5):223–32 (in German).

Khan, M.A., "Nutritional therapy of the patient with diabetes mellitus. Abstract." *J Am Coll Nutr,* 1994; 13(5):520.

Maki, K.C., et al., "Fiber intake and risk of developing non-insulin-dependent diabetes mellitus." Letter. *JAMA,* 1997; 277(22):1761.

McCarty, M.F., "Toward a wholly nutritional therapy for type 2 diabetes." *Med Hypotheses,* 2000; 54:483–7.

McCarty, M.F., "Toward practical prevention of type 2 diabetes." *Med Hypotheses,* 2000; 54:786–93.

Meyer, K.A., Kushi, L.H., Jacobs, D.R. Jr., et al., "Carbohydrates, dietary fiber, and incident type 2 diabetes in older women." *Am J Clin Nutr,* 2000; 71:921–30.

O'Dea, K., "Marked improvement in carbohydrate and lipid metabolism in diabetic Australian aborigines after temporary reversion to traditional lifestyle." *Diabetes,* 1984; 33(6):596–603.

Raal, F.J., et al., "Effect of moderate protein restriction on the progression of overt diabetic nephropathy: a 6-mo prospective study." *Am J Clin Nutr,* 1994; 60:579–85.

Reaven, G.M., :Dietary therapy for non-insulin-dependent diabetes mellitus." Editorial. *N Engl J Med.* 1988; 319(13):862–64.

Ryan, E.A., Pick, M.E., Marceau, C., "Use of alternative medicines in diabetes mellitus." *Diabet Med,* 2001; 18:242–5.

Salmeron, J., Hu, F.B., Manson, J.E., et al., "Dietary fat intake and risk of type 2 diabetes in women." *Am J Clin Nutr,* 2001; 73:1019–26.

Schmidt, L.E., et al., "Evaluation of nutrient intake in subjects with non-insulin-dependent diabetes mellitus." *J Am Diet Assoc,* 1994; 94(7):773–4.

Schmidt, L.E., et al., "Evaluation of nutrient intake in subjects with non-insulin-dependent diabetes mellitus." *J Am Diet Assoc,* 1994; 94(7):773–4.

Singh, R.B., et al., "Dietary intake and plasma levels of antioxidant vitamins in health and disease: a hospital-based case-control study." *J Nutr Environ Med,* 1995; 5:235–42.

Snowdon, D.A., Phillips, R.L., "Does a vegetarian diet reduce the occurrence of diabetes?" *Am J Public Health,* 1995; 75(5):507–12.

Straub, R.H., et al., "No evidence of deficiency A, E, beta-carotene, B1, B2, B6, B12 and folate in neuropathic non-insulin-dependent diabetic women." *Int J Vitam Nutr Res,* 1993; 63(3):239–40.

Tuomilehto, J., Lindstrom, J., Eriksson, J.G., et al., "Finnish Diabetes Prevention Study Group. Prevention of type 2 diabetes mellitus by changes in lifestyle among subjects with impaired glucose tolerance." *N Engl J Med,* 2001; 344:1343–50.

Williams, G., "Management of non-insulin-dependent diabetes mellitus." *Lancet,* 1994; 343:95–100.

CHROMIUM

"Chromium supplementation decreases cardiac risk in diabetics, Intern Med World Rep." *Am Heart J,* July 2005; 149:632–636.

Albarracin, C.A., Fuqua, B.C., et al., "Chromium picolinate and biotin combination improves glucose metabolism in treated, uncontrolled overweight to obese patients with type 2 diabetes." *Diabetes Metab Res Rev,* 2008; 24(1): 41–51.

Anderson, R., "Chromium in the prevention and control of diabetes." *Diabetes and Metabolism (Paris),* 2000; 26(1):22–27.

Anderson, R.A., et al., "Elevated intakes of supplemental chromium improve glucose and insulin variables in individuals with type 2 diabetes." *Diabetes,* 1997; 46(11):1786–91.

Anderson, R.A., "Chromium, glucose intolerance and diabetes." *J Am Coll Nutr,* 1998; 17(6):548–555.

Anderson, R.A., "Chromium, glucose tolerance, and diabetes." *Biol Trace Elem Res,* 1992; 32:19–24.

Bahijiri, S.M., Mira, S.A., Mufti, A.M., et al., "The effects of inorganic chromium and brewer's yeast supplementation on glucose tolerance, serum lipids and drug dosage in individuals with type 2 diabetes." *Saudi Med J,* 2000; 21:831–7.

Cefalu, W.T., Rood, J., et al., "Characterization of the metabolic and physiologic response to chromium supplementation in subjects with type 2 diabetes mellitus." *Metabolism,* 2009

Davies, D.M., et al., "The isolation of glucose tolerance factors from brewer's yeast and their relationship to chromium." *Biochem Med,* 1985; 33(3):297–311.

Finney, L.S., Gonzalez-Campoy, M., "Dietary chromium and diabetes: is there a relationship?" *Clin Diabetes,* 1997; 15(1).

Freund, H., et al., "Chromium deficiency during total parenteral nutrition." *JAMA,* 1979; 241(5):496-8.

Geohas, J., Daly, A., et al., "Chromium picolinate and biotin combination reduces atherogenic index of plasma in patients with type 2 diabetes mellitus: a placebo-controlled, double-blinded, randomized clinical trial." *American Journal of the Medical Sciences,* 2007; 333(3): 145-153.

Haylock, S.J., et al., "Separation of biologically active chromium-containing complexes from yeast extracts and other sources of glucose tolerance factor (GTF) activity." *J Inorg Biochem,* 1983; 18(3):195-211.

Jeejeebhoy, K.N., et al., "Chromium deficiency, glucose tolerance, and neuropathy reversed by chromium supplementation, in a patient receiving long-term parenteral nutrition." *Am J Clin Nutr,* 1977; 30(4):531-8.

Jovanovic-Petersen. L., et al., "Chromium supplementation for gestational diabetic women improves glucose tolerance and decreases hyperinsulinemia. Abstract." *J Am Coll Nutr,* 1995; 14(5):530.

Kazi, T.G., Afridi, H.I., et al., "Copper, chromium, manganese, iron, nickel, and zinc levels in biological samples of diabetes mellitus patients." *Biol Trace Elem Res,* 2008; 122(1): 1-18.

Kleefstra, N., Houweling, S.T., et al., "Chromium treatment has no effect in patients with poorly controlled, insulin-treated type 2 diabetes in an obese Western population: a randomized, double-blind, placebo-controlled trial." *Diabetes Care,* 2006; 29(3): 521-5.

Kozlovsky, A.S., et al., "Effects of diets high in simple sugars on urinary chromium losses." *Metabolism,* 1986; 35(6):515-18.

Liu, V.J., Abernathy, R.P., "Chromium and insulin in young subjects with normal glucose tolerance." *Am J Clin Nutr,* 1982; 25(4):661-7.

Martin, J., Wang, Z.Q., et al., "Chromium picolinate supplementation attenuates body weight gain and increases insulin sensitivity in subjects with type 2 diabetes." *Diabetes Care,* 2006; 29(8):1826-32.

Mertz, W., "Chromium occurrence and function in a biological system." *Physiol Rev,* 1969; 49:163-230.

Mertz, W., "Effects and metabolism of glucose tolerance factor." *Nutr Rev,* 1975; 33(5):129-35.

Offenbacher, E., Stunyer, F., "Beneficial effect of chromium-rich yeast on glucose tolerance and blood lipids in elderly patients." *Diabetes,* 1980; 29:919-25.

Pei, D., Hsieh, C.H., et al., "The influence of chromium chloride-containing milk to glycemic control of patients with type 2 diabetes mellitus: a randomized, double-blind, placebo-controlled trial." *Metabolism,* 2006; 55(7):923-7.

Racek, J., Trefil, L., et al., "Influence of chromium-enriched yeast on blood glucose and insulin variables, blood lipids, and markers of oxidative stress in subjects with type 2 diabetes mellitus." *Biol Trace Elem Res,* 2006; 109(3):215-30.

Ravina, A., et al., "Reversal of corticosteroid-induced diabetes mellitus with supplemental chromium." *Diabet Med,* 1999; 16:164-167.

Simonoff, M., et al., "The isolation of glucose tolerance factors from brewer's yeast and their relation to chromium." *Biol Trace Elem Res*, 1992; 32:25–8.

Singer, G.M., Geohas, J., "The effect of chromium picolinate and biotin supplementation on glycemic control in poorly controlled patients with type 2 diabetes mellitus: a placebo-controlled, double-blinded, randomized trial." *Diabetes Technol Ther*, 2006, 8(6):636–643.

Vrtovec, M., Vrtovec, B., et al., "Chromium supplementation shortens QTc interval duration in patients with type 2 diabetes mellitus." *Am Heart J*, 2005; 149:632–636.

MAGNESIUM

"Dietary magnesium and fiber intakes and inflammatory and metabolic indicators in middle-aged subjects from a population-based cohort." *Am J Clin Nutr*, 2006; 84(5):1062–9.

"Magnesium and Diabetes." *Practical Diabetology*, March/April 1991; 10(2):1–5.

American Diabetes Association. Consensus panel. "Magnesium supplementation in the treatment of diabetes." *Diabetes Care*, 1995; 18(Suppl 1):83–5.

American Diabetes Association. Consensus statement. "Magnesium supplementation in the treatment of diabetes." *Diabetes Care*, 1992; 15(8):1065–7.

Balon, Thomas, W., et al., "Dietary magnesium prevents fructose-induced insulin insensitivity in rats." *Hypertension*, June 1994; 23(6) Part II:1036–1039.

Bartlett, H.E., Eperjesi, F., "Nutritional supplementation for type 2 diabetes: a systematic review." *Ophthalmic Physiol Opt*, 2008; 28(6):503–23.

Colditz, G.A., et al., "Diet and risk of clinical diabetes in women." *Am J Clin Nutr*, 1992; 55:1018–23.

Corica, F., et al., "Magnesium levels in plasma, erythrocyte, and platelets in hypertensive and normotensive patients with non-insulin-dependent diabetes mellitus." *Biol trace Elem Res*, 1996; 51:130–2.

Corica, F., Corsonello, A., et al., "Serum ionized magnesium levels in relation to metabolic syndrome in type 2 diabetic patients." *J Am Coll Nutr*, 2006; 25(3):210–5.

deLourdes, Lima, M., et al., "The effect of magnesium supplementation in increasing doses on the control of type 2 diabetes." *Diabetes Care*, May 1998; 21(5):682–686.

Djurhuus, M.S., Klitgaard, N.A., Pedersen, K.K., et al., "Magnesium reduces insulin-stimulated glucose uptake and serum lipid concentrations in type 1 diabetes." *Metabolism*, 2001; 50:1409–17.

Eibl, N.L., et al., "Hypomagnesemia in non-insulin-dependent diabetes: effect of a 3-month replacement therapy." *Diabetes Care*, 1995; 18(2):188–92.

Elamin, A., Tuvemo, T., "Magnesium and insulin-dependent diabetes mellitus." *Diabetes Res Clin Pract*, 1990; 10:203–9.

Elamin, Abdelaziz and Tuvemo, Torsten, "Magnesium and insulin-dependent diabetes mellitus." *Diabetes Research and Clinical Practice*, 1990; 10:203–209.

Farvid, M.S., Jalali, M., et al., "Comparison of the effects of vitamins and/or mineral supplementation on glomerular and tubular dysfunction in type 2 diabetes." *Diabetes Care*, 2005; 28(10):2458–2464.

Hadjistavri, L.S., Sarafidis, P.A., et al., "Beneficial effects of oral magnesium supplementation on insulin sensitivity and serum lipid profile." *Med Sci Monit*, 2010; 16(6):PI13–18.

He, K., Liu, K., et al., "Magnesium intake and incidence of metabolic syndrome among young adults." *Circulation,* 2006, Vol. 113.

Head, K.A., "Peripheral neuropathy: pathogenic mechanisms and alternative therapies." *Altern Med Rev,* 2006; 11(4):294–329.

Huerta, M.G., Roemmich, J.N., et al., "Magnesium deficiency is associated with insulin resistance in obese children." *Diabetes Care,* 2005; 28(5):1175–81.

Lostroh, A.J., Krahl, "Magnesium, a second messenger for insulin: Ion translocation coupled to transport activity." *Adv Enz Regul,* 1974; 12:73–81.

Ma, J., et al., "Associations of serum and dietary magnesium with cardiovascular disease, hypertension, diabetes, insulin and carotid artery wall thickness: the ARIC study." *J Clin Epidemiol,* 1995; 48(7):927–40.

McNair, P., et al., "Hypomagnesemia, a risk factor for diabetic retinopathy." *Diabetes,* 1978; 27:1075–7.

Mooren, F.C., Kraus, A., et al., "Oral magnesium supplementation reduces insulin resistance in non-diabetic subjects - a double-blind, placebo-controlled, randomized trial." *Diabetes Obes Metab,* Nov 18 2010.

Nadler, J.L., et al., "Magnesium deficiency produces insulin resistance and increased thromboxane synthesis." *Hypertension,* 1993; 21:1024–9.

Ohira, T., Peacock, J.M., et al., "Serum and dietary magnesium and risk of ischemic stroke: The atherosclerosis risk in communities study." *Am J Epidemiol,* April 16 2009.

Paolisso, G., et al., "Improved insulin response and action by chronic magnesium administration in aged NIDDM subjects." *Diabetes Care,* 1989; 12:265–69.

Pham, P.C.T., Pham, P.M.T., et al., "Lower serum magnesium levels are associated with more rapid decline of renal function in patients with diabetes mellitus type 2." *Clin Nephrol,* 2005;63(6):429–436.

Purvis, John R., M.D., et al., "Effect of oral magnesium supplementation on selected cardiovascular risk factors in non-insulin-dependent diabetics." Archives of *Family Medicine,* June 1994; 3:503–508.

Rodriguez-Moran, M., Guerrero-Romero, F., "Oral magnesium supplementation improves insulin sensitivity and metabolic control in type 2 diabetic subjects: A randomized double-blind controlled trial." *Diabetes Care,* April 2003; 26(4):1147–1152.

Rumawas, M.E., McKeown, N.M., et al., "Magnesium intake is related to improved insulin homeostasis in the Framingham offspring cohort." *Journal of the American College of Nutrition,* 2006; 25(6):486–92.

Sjogren, A., et al., "Magnesium potassium and zinc deficiency in subjects with type II diabetes mellitus." *Acta Med Scand,* 1988; 224:461–3.

Soltani, N., Keshavarz, M., et al., "Effects of administration of oral magnesium on plasma glucose and pathological changes in the aorta and pancreas of diabetic rats." *Clin Exp Pharmacol Physiol,* 2005; 32(8):604–10.

Song, Y., Li, T.Y., et al., "Magnesium intake and plasma concentrations of markers of systemic inflammation and endothelial dysfunction in women." *Am J Clin Nutr,* 2007; 85(4):1068–74.

Tosiello, L., "Hypomagnesemia and diabetes mellitus." *Arch Intern Med,* 1996; 156:1143–8.

van Dam, R.M., Hu, F.B., et al., "Dietary calcium and magnesium, major food sources, and risk of type 2 diabetes in U.S. black women." *Diabetes Care*, 2006; 29(10):2238–43.

Villegas, R., Gao, Y.T., et al., "Dietary calcium and magnesium intakes and the risk of type 2 diabetes: the Shanghai Women's Health Study." *J Clin Nutr*, 2009; 89(4):1059–67.

Wen-Gang, Z., et al., "Hypomagnesemia and heart complications in diabetes mellitus." *Chin Med J*, 1987; 100:719–22.

Wimhurst, J.M., Manchester, K.L., "Comparison of ability of Mg and Mn to activate the key enzymes of glycolysis." *FEBS Letters*, 1972; 27:321–6.

Wolk, A., "Magnesium intake and risk of type 2 diabetes: a meta-analysis." Larsson SC, *J Intern Med*, 2007; 262(2):208–14.

ZINC

Andrews, R.C., Richardson, "Diabetes and schizophrenia: Genes or zinc deficiency?" *The Lancet*, November 7, 1992; 340:1160.

Bartlett, H.E., Eperjesi, F., "Nutritional supplementation for type 2 diabetes: a systematic review." *Ophthalmic Physiol Opt*, 2008; 28(6):503–23.

Bonnefont-Rousselot, D., "The role of antioxidant micronutrients in the prevention of diabetic complications." *Treat Endocrinol*, 2004; 3(1):41–52.

Brun, J.F., et al., "Effects of oral zinc gluconate on glucose effectiveness and insulin sensitivity in humans." *Biol Trace Elem Res*, 1995; 47:385–91.

Chausmer, A.B., "Zinc, insulin and diabetes." *J Am Coll Nutr*, 1998; 17(2).

Cunningham, J.J., et al., "Hyperzincuria in individuals with insulin-dependent diabetes mellitus: concurrent zinc status and the effect of high-dose zinc supplementation." *Metabolism*, 1994; 43:1558–62.

Farvid, M.S., Jalali, M., et al., "Comparison of the effects of vitamins and/or mineral supplementation on glomerular and tubular dysfunction in type 2 diabetes." *Diabetes Care*, 2005; 28(10):2458–2464.

Haglund, B., et al., "Evidence of a relationship between childhood-onset type I diabetes and low groundwater concentration of zinc." *Diabetes Care*, 1996; 19(8):873–5.

Heidarian, E., Amini, M., et al., "Effect of zinc supplementation on serum homocysteine in type 2 diabetic patients with microalbuminuria." *Rev Diabet Stud*, 2009; 6(1):64–70.

Kadhim, H.M., Ismail, S.H., et al., "Effects of melatonin and zinc on lipid profile and renal function in type 2 diabetic patients poorly controlled with metformin." *Pineal Res*, 2006; 41(2):189–193.

Kinlaw, W.B., et al., "Abnormal zinc metabolism in type II diabetes mellitus." *Am J Med*, 1983; 75(2):273–7.

Marchesini, G., et al., "Zinc Supplementation Improves Glucose Disposal in Patients With Cirrhosis." *Metabolism*, July 1998; 47(7):792–798.

Mateo, M.C., et al., "Serum zinc, copper and insulin in diabetes mellitus." *Biomedicine*, 1978; 29(2):56–8.

McNair, P., et al., "Hyperzincuria in insulin treated diabetes mellitus: Its relation to glucose homeostasis and insulin administration." *Clin Chim Acta*, 1981; 112:343–8.

O'Keefe, J.H., Jr, Cordain, L., "Cardiovascular disease resulting from a diet and lifestyle at odds with our paleolithic genome: How to become a 21st-century hunter-gatherer." *Mayo Clin Proc,* January 2004; 79:101–108.

Parham, M., Heidarian, E., et al., "Effect of zinc supplementation on microalbuminuria in patients with type 2 diabetes: a double blind, randomized, placebo-controlled, cross-over trial." *Rev Diabet Stud,* 2008; 5(2): 102–9.

Raz, I., et al., "The influence of zinc supplementation on glucose homeostasis in NIDDM." *Diabetes Res,* 1989; 11(2):73–9.

Roussel, A-M., Kerkeni, A., et al., "Antioxidant effects of zinc supplementation in Tunisians with type 2 diabetes mellitus." *J Am Coll Nutr,* 2003; 22(4):316–321.

Salgueiro, M.J., Krebs, N., Zubillaga, M.B., et al., "Zinc and diabetes mellitus: Is there a need of zinc supplementation in diabetes mellitus patients?" *Biol Trace Elem Res,* 2001; 81:215–228.

Shidfar, F., Aghasi, M., et al., "Effects of combination of zinc and vitamin A supplementation on serum fasting blood sugar, insulin, apoprotein B and apoprotein A-I in patients with type I diabetes." *Int J Food Sci Nutr,* 2010; 61(2): 182–91.

Sjogren, A., et al., "Magnesium potassium and zinc deficiency in subjects with type II diabetes mellitus." *Acta Med Scand,* 1988; 224:461–3.

Soinio, M., Marniemi, J., et al., "Serum zinc level and coronary heart disease events in patients with type 2 diabetes." *Diabetes Care,* 2007; 30(3):523–8.

Solomon, S.J., King, J.C., "Effect of low zinc intake on carbohydrate and fat metabolism in men." *Fed Proc,* 1983; 42:391.

Solomons, N.W., "On the assessment of zinc and copper nutriture in man." *Am J Clin Nutr,* 1979; 32:856–71.

Sun, Q., Hu, F.B., et al., "A prospective study of zinc intake and risk of type 2 diabetes in women." *Diabetes Care,* Jan 26, 2009.

VANADIUM

Badmaev, V., et al., "Vanadium: A review of its potential role in the fight against diabetes." *J Altern Complement Med,* 1999; 5(3):273–291.

Brichard, S.M., Henquin, J.C., "The role of vanadium in the management of diabetes." *Trends Pharmacol Sci,* 1995; 16(8):265–70.

Cusi, K., Cukier, S., DeFronzo, R.A., et al., "Vanadyl sulfate improves hepatic and muscle insulin sensitivity in type 2 diabetes." *J Clin Endocrinol Metab,* 2001; 86(3):1410–1417.

Domingo, J.L., et al., "Oral vanadium administration to streptozotocin-diabetic rats has marked negative side-effects which are independent of the form of vanadium used." *Toxicology,* 1991; 66:279–87.

Domingo, J.L., "Vanadium and diabetes. What about vanadium toxicity?" *Mol Cell Biochem,* 2000; 203:185–187.

French, Rodney, J., and Jones, Peter, J., "Role of vanadium in nutrition: Metabolism, essentiality and dietary considerations." *Life Sciences,* 1993; 52(4):339–346.

Halberstam, M., "Oral vanadyl sulfate improves insulin sensitivity in NIDDM but not in obese diabetic subjects." *Diabetes,* 1996; 45:659–66.

Lind, L. et al., "Relation of serum calcium concentration to metabolic risk factors for cardiovascular disease." *Br Med J,* 1988; 297:960–3.

Thompson, K.H., Orvig, C., "Vanadium compounds in the treatment of diabetes." *Met Ions Biol Syst*, 2004; 41:7:221–252.

Verma, Subodh, Ph.D., et al., "Nutritional factors that can favorably influence the glucose/insulin system: Vanadium." *Journal of the American College of Nutrition*, 1998; 17(1):11–18.

CALCIUM

De Fronzo, R.A., Lang, R., "Hypophosphatemia and glucose intolerance: Evidence for tissue insensitivity to insulin." *N Engl J Med*, 1980; 303(22):1259–63.

Fogh-Andersen, N., et al., "Lowered serum ionized calcium in insulin treated diabetic subjects." *Scand J Clin Lab Invest Suppl*, 1983; 165:93–7.

Fujita, T., et al., "Insulin secretion after oral calcium load." *Endocrinol Jpn*, 1978; 25(6):645–8.

Kawagishi, T., et al., "Calcium metabolism in diabetes mellitus." *J Nutr Sci Vitaminol (Tokyo)*, 1991; 37 Suppl:S51-S56.

Levy, J., et al., "Diabetes mellitus: a disease of abnormal cellular calcium metabolism?" *Am J Med*, 1994; 260–71.

Sanchez, M., "Oral calcium supplementation reduces intraplatelet free calcium concentration and insulin resistance in essential hypertensive patients." *Hypertension*, 1992; 29(2):531–6.

POTASSIUM

Durlach, J., Collery, P., "Magnesium and potassium in diabetes and carbohydrate metabolism. Review of the present status and recent results." *Magnesium*, 1984; 3(4–6):315–23.

Greene, D.A., et al., "Are disturbances of sorbitol, phosphoinositide, and Na+-K+=-ATPase regulation involved in pathogenesis of diabetic neuropathy?" *Diabetes*.

Norbiato, G., et al., "Effects of potassium supplementation on insulin binding and insulin action in human obesity: Protein-modified fast and refeeding." *Europe J Clin Invest*, 1984; 44:414–9.

Perez, G.O., et al., "Potassium homeostasis in chronic diabetes mellitus." *Arch Intern Med*, 1977: 137(8):1018–22.

Sjogren, A., et al., "Magnesium potassium and zinc deficiency in subjects with type II diabetes mellitus." *Acta Med Scand*, 1988; 224:461–3.

MANGANESE

Baly, D., et al., "Effect of manganese deficiency on insulin binding, glucose transport and metabolism of rat adipocytes." *J Nutr*, 1990; 120:1075–9.

Rubenstein, A.H.. "Hypoglycemia induced by manganese." *Nature*, 1962; 194:188–89.

Wimhurst, J.M., Manchester, K.L., "Comparison of ability of Mg and Mn to activate the key enzymes of glycolysis." *FEBS Letters*, 1972; 27:321–6.

COPPER

Fields, M., et al., "Accumulation of sorbitol in copper deficiency: Dependency on gender and type of dietary carbohydrate." *Metabolism*, 1989: 38(4):371–75.

Klevey, L.M., et al., "Diminished glucose tolerance in two men to a diet low in copper." *Am J Clin Nutr,* 1983; 37:717.

Reiser, S., et al., "Indices of copper status in humans consuming a typical American diet containing either fructose or starch." *Am J Clin Nutr,* 1985; 42:242–51.

Solomons, N.W.. "On the assessment of zinc and copper nutriture in man." *Am J Clin Nutr,* 1979; 32:856–71.

VITAMIN C

Afkhami-Ardekani, M., Shojaoddiny-Ardekani, A., et al., "Effect of vitamin C on blood glucose, serum lipids & serum insulin in type 2 diabetes patients." *Indian J Med Res,* 2007; 126(5):471–4.

Aladag, I., Erkokmaz, U., et al., "Role of oxidative stress in hearing impairment in patients with type two diabetes mellitus." *J Laryngol Otol,* 2009; 123(9):957–63.

Azadbakht, L., Esmaillzadeh, A., "Dietary and non-dietary determinants of central adiposity among Tehrani women." *Public Health Nutr,* 2007; 1–7.

Banerjee, S.. "Physiological role of dehydroascorbic acid." *Indian J Physiol Pharmacol,* 1977; 21(2):85–93.

Birlouez-Aragon, I., Delcourt, C., Tessier, F., Papoz, L., "Associations of Age, Smoking Habits and Diabetes With Plasma Vitamin C of Elderly of the POLA Study." *Int J Vitam Nutr Res,* 2001;71(1):53–59.

Block, G., Jensen, C.D., et al., "Usage patterns, health, and nutritional status of long-term multiple dietary supplement users: a cross-sectional study." *Nutr J,* 2007; 6(1):30.

Ceriello, A., Kumar, S., et al., "Simultaneous control of hyperglycemia and oxidative stress normalizes endothelial function in type 1 diabetes." *Diabetes Care,* 2007; 30(3):649–654.

Chui, M.H., Greenwood, C.E., "Antioxidant vitamins reduce acute meal-induced memory deficits in adults with type 2 diabetes." *Nutrition Research,* 2008; 28(7):423–429.

Clemetson, A.B.. "Ascorbic acid and diabetes mellitus." *Med Hypotheses,* 1976; 2:193–4.

Cogan, D.G., et al., "Aldose reductase and complications of diabetes." *Ann Intem Med,* 1984; 101:82–91.

Cox, B.D., Butterfield, W.J.H., "Vitamin C supplements and diabetic cutaneous capillary fragility." *Br Med J,* 1975; 3:205.

Cunningham, J.J., et al., "Reduced mononuclear leukocyte ascorbic-acid content in adults with insulin-dependent diabetes mellitus consuming adequate dietary vitamin C." *Metabolism,* 1991; 40:146–9.

Cunningham, J.J., et al., "Vitamin C: an aldose reductase inhibitor that normalizes erythrocyte sorbitol in insulin-dependent diabetes mellitus." *J Am Coll Nutr,* 1994; 13(4):344–50.

Cunningham, J.J., "The glucose/insulin system and vitamin C: implications in insulin-dependent diabetes mellitus." *J Am Coll Nutr,* 1998; 17(2):105–8.

Cunningham, John, J., Ph.D., "The glucose/insulin system and vitamin C: Implications in insulin-dependent diabetes mellitus." *Journal of the American College of Nutrition,* 1998; 17(2):105–108.

Davison, G.W., Ashton, T., et al., "Molecular detection of exercise-induced free radicals following ascorbate prophylaxis in type 1 diabetes mellitus: a randomized controlled trial." *Diabetologia*, September 4, 2008.

Dice, J.F., Denial, C.W., "The hypoglycemic effect of ascorbic acid in a juvenile-onset diabetic." *J Int Res Commun*, 1973; 1(1):41.

Ditzel, J., "Oxygen transport in diabetes." *Diabetes*, 1976; 25:832–8.

Eriksson, J., Kohvakka, A., "Magnesium and ascorbic acid supplementation in diabetes mellitus." *Ann Nutr Metab*, 1995; 39(4):217–23.

Farvid, M.S., Jalali, M., et al., "Comparison of the effects of vitamins and/or mineral supplementation on glomerular and tubular dysfunction in type 2 diabetes." *Diabetes Care*, 2005; 28(10):2458–2464.

Gaede, P., Poulsen, H,E., et al., "Double-blind, randomized study of the effect of combined treatment with vitamin C and E on albuminuria in type 2 diabetic patients." *Diabet Med*, 2001;18:756–760.

Gaede, P., Poulsen, H.E., Parving, H.H., et al., "Double-blind, randomized study of the effect of combined treatment with vitamin C and E on albuminuria in type 2 diabetic patients." *Diabet Med*, 2001; 18:756–60.

Ginter, E., et al., "Hypocholesterolemic effect of ascorbic acid in maturity-onset diabetes mellitus." *Int J Vitam Nutr Res*, 1978; 48(4):368–73.

Ginter, E.M., "Chorvathova V. Vitamin C and diabetes mellitus." *Nutr Health*, 1983; 2:3–11.

Harding, A.H., Wareham, N.J., et al., "Plasma vitamin C level, fruit and vegetable consumption, and the risk of new-onset type 2 diabetes mellitus: The European Prospective Investigation of Cancer-Norfolk Prospective Study." *Arch Intern Med*, 2008; 168(14):1493–1499.

Jaspan, J., et al., "Treatment of severely painful diabetic neuropathy with an aldose reductase inhibitor: Relief of pain and improved somatic and autonomic nerve function." *Lancet*, 1983; 2:758–62.

Jaxa-Chamiec, T., Bednarz, B., et al., "Effects of vitamins C and E on the outcome after acute myocardial infarction in diabetics: A Retrospective, Hypothesis-Generating Analysis from the MIVIT Study." *Cardiology*, 2008; 112(3):219–223.

Jennings, P.E. et al., "Vitamin C metabolites and microangiopathy in diabetes mellitus." *Diabetes Res*, 1987; 6(3):151–4.

Jin, Y., Cui, X., et al., "Systemic inflammatory load in humans is suppressed by consumption of two formulations of dried, encapsulated juice concentrate." *Mol Nutr Food Res*, April 27, 2010.

Kapeghian, J.C., Verlangieri, A.J., "The effects of glucose on ascorbic acid uptake in heart endothelial cells: Possible pathogenesis of diabetic angiopathies." *Life Sci*, 1984; 34(6):577–84.

Neri, S., Signorelli, S.S., et al., "Effects of antioxidant supplementation on postprandial oxidative stress and endothelial dysfunction: A single-blind, 15-day clinical trial in patients with untreated type 2 diabetes, subjects with impaired glucose tolerance, and healthy controls." *Clin Ther*, 2005; 27(11):1764–73.

Odermarsky, M., Lykkesfeldt, J., et al., "Poor vitamin C status is associated with increased carotid intima-media thickness, decreased microvascular function, and delayed myocardial repolarization in young patients with type 1 diabetes." *Am J Clin Nutr*, June 24, 2009.

Padayatty, S.J., Sun, A.Y., et al., "Vitamin C: intravenous use by complementary and alternative medicine practitioners and adverse effects." *PLoS One*, 2010; 5(7):e11414.

Patterson, J.W., "The diabetogenic effect of dehydroascorbic acid and dehydroisoascorbic acids." *J Bio Chem*, 1950; 183:81.

Rizzo, M.R., Abbatecola, A.M., et al., "Evidence for anti-inflammatory effects of combined administration of vitamin E and C in older persons with impaired fasting glucose: impact on insulin action." *J Am Coll Nutr*, 2008; 27(4):505–11.

Sinclair, A.J., et al., "Low plasma ascorbate levels in patients with type 2 diabetes mellitus consuming adequate dietary vitamin C." *Diabetic Med*, 1994; 11:893–8.

Som, S., et al., "Ascorbic acid metabolism in diabetes mellitus." *Metabolism*, 1981; 30(6):572–7.

Tessier, D.M., Khalil, A., et al., "Effects of vitamin C supplementation on antioxidants and lipid peroxidation markers in elderly subjects with type 2 diabetes." *Arch Gerontol Geriatr*, Dec 10, 2007.

Vinson, J.A., Howard, T.B., III., "Inhibition of protein glycation and advanced glycation end products by ascorbic acid and other vitamins and nutrients." *J Nutr Biochem*, 1996; 7:659–63.

Wannamethee, S.G., Lowe, G.D., et al., "Associations of vitamin C status, fruit and vegetable intakes, and markers of inflammation and hemostasis." *Am J Clin Nutr*, 2006; 83(3):567–74.

Will, J.C., Byers, T., "Does diabetes mellitus increase the requirement for vitamin C?" *Nutr Rev*, 1996; 54(7):193–202.

Williams, M.A., et al., "Vitamin C and the risk of gestational diabetes mellitus: A Case-control Study," *J Reprod Med*, April 2004;49(4):257–266.

Yamada, H., Waki, M., et al., "Lymphocyte and plasma vitamin C levels in type 2 diabetic patients with and without diabetes complications." *Diabetes Care*, October 2004; 27(10):2491–2492.

Zebrowski, E.J., Bhatnagar, P.K., "Urinary excretion pattern of ascorbic acid in streptozotocin diabetic and insulin treated rats." *Pharm Res Commun*, 1979; 11(2):95–103.

THE VITAMIN B COMPLEX

Block, G., Jensen, C.D., et al., "Usage patterns, health, and nutritional status of long-term multiple dietary supplement users: a cross-sectional study." *Nutr J*, 2007; 6(1):30.

Chernoff, Ronni, Ph.D., RD, "Pharmacology, nutrition, and the elderly: Interaction and implications," Suter, Paolo and Blumberg, Jeffrey B., Chapter 13;337–361/Geriatric Nutrition, The Professional's Handbook, Aspen Publication, Aspen Publishers, Inc., Gathersburg, MD 1991.

Deshmukh, U.S., Joglekar, C.V., et al., "Effect of physiological doses of oral vitamin B(12) on plasma homocysteine: a randomized, placebo-controlled, double-blind trial in India." *European Journal of Clinical Nutrition*, March 10, 2010.

Jolivalt, C.G., Mizisin, L.M., et al., "B vitamins alleviate indices of neuropathic pain in diabetic rats." *Eur J Pharmacol*, 2009; 612(1–3):41–7.

Krishnaveni, G.V., Hill, J.C., et al., "Low plasma vitamin B(12) in pregnancy is associated with gestational 'diabesity' and later diabetes." *Diabetologia*, Aug 26, 2009.

Levy, Y., Yeromenko, Y., et al., "B-group vitamins reduce plasma homocysteine concentration in patients with type 2 diabetes mellitus and normal basal homocysteine." *J Nutr Environ Med*, June 2003;13(2):79–85.

Murphy-Chutorian, Douglas, M.D., Alderman, Edwin L., M.D., "The case that hyperhomocysteinemia is a risk factor for coronary artery disease." *The American Journal of Cardiology*, April 1, 1994;73:705–706.

Pflipsen, M., Oh, R.C., et al., "The prevalence of vitamin B(12) deficiency in patients with type 2 diabetes: a cross-sectional study." *J Am Board Fam Med*, 2009; 22(5):528–34.

Rieder, H.P., et al., "Vitamin status in diabetic neuropathy (thiamine, riboflavin, pyridoxine, cobalamin and tocopherol)." *Z Emahrungswiss*, 1980; 19(1):1–13.

Shen, J., Lai, C.Q., et al., "Association of vitamin B-6 status with inflammation, oxidative stress, and chronic inflammatory conditions: the Boston Puerto Rican Health Study." *Am J Clin Nutr*, Dec 2, 2009.

Stracke, H., et al, "A benfotiamine-vitamin B combination in treatment of diabetic polyneuropathy," *Experimental and Clinical Endocrinology and Diabetes*, 1996; 104:311–316.

Ting, R.Z., Szeto, C.C., et al., "Risk factors of vitamin B(12) deficiency in patients receiving metformin." *Arch Intern Med*, 2006; 166(18):1975–9.

Yajnik, C.S., Deshpande, S.S., et al., "Vitamin B(12) and folate concentrations during pregnancy and insulin resistance in the offspring: the Pune Maternal Nutrition Study." *Diabetologia*, 2008; 51(1):29–38.

VITAMIN B1 THIAMINE

Al-Fawaz, Ibrahim, M., M.D., et al., "Annals - Thiamine dependent anemia and DIDMOAD (WOLFRAM) syndrome: Further studies and report of two additional cases," *Saudi Medicine*, 1992; 12(3):309–312.

Alzahrani, A.S., Baitei, E., et al., "Thiamine transporter mutation: an example of monogenic diabetes mellitus." *European Journal of Endocrinology*, 2006; 155(6):787–792.

Arora, S., Lidor, A., et al., "Thiamine (vitamin B1) improves endothelium-dependent vasodilatation in the presence of hyperglycemia." *Ann Vasc Surg*, 2006; 20(5):653–8.

Evans, D.I.K., "Thiamine response of anemia." *British Journal of Hematology*, 1991; 78:140–141.

Neufeld, E.J., Fleming, J.C., Tartaglini, E., Steinkamp, M.P., "Thiamine-responsive megaloblastic anemia syndrome: A disorder of high-affinity thiamine transport." *Blood Cells Mol Dis*, February 2001; 27(1):135–138.

Rabbani, N., Alam, S.S., et al., "High-dose thiamine therapy for patients with type 2 diabetes and microalbuminuria: a randomized, double-blind placebo-controlled pilot study." *Diabetologia*, Dec 5, 2008.

Saito, N. et al., "Blood thiamine levels in outpatients with diabetes mellitus." *J Nutr Sci Vitaminol (Tokyo)*, 1987; 33(6):421–30.

Skelton, W.P., III, Skelton, N.K., "Thiamine deficiency neuropathy: It's still common today." *Postgrad Med*, 1989; 85(8):301–6.

Stracke, H., et al., "A benfotiamine-vitamin B combination in treatment of diabetic polyneuropathy." *Exp Clin Endocrinol Diabetes*, 1996; 104(4):311–16.

Thornalley, P.J., Bodmer, C.W., et al., "High prevalence of low plasma thiamine concentration in diabetes linked to a marker of vascular disease." *Diabetologia*, August 4, 2007.

Wu, S., Ren, J., "Benfotiamine alleviates diabetes-induced cerebral oxidative damage independent of advanced glycation end-product, tissue factor and TNF-alpha." *Neurosci Lett*, 2006; 394(2):158–162.

VITAMIN B2 RIBOFLAVIN

Blumberg, J., "The requirement for vitamins in aging and age-associated degenerative conditions." *Vitamin Intake in Human Nutrition*, Basel, Karger, 1995; 52:108–115.

Garland, Donita L., "Ascorbic acid and the eye," *American Journal of Clinical Nutrition*, 1991; 54:1198S–1202S.

Sandyk, Reuven, "L-Tryptophan in neuropsychiatric disorders: A review." *International Journal of Neuroscience*, 1992; 67:127–144.

VITAMIN B3 NIACIN OR NIACINAMIDE

"Niacin for dyslipidemia in diabetes: Not such a bad idea?" *Emergency Med*, July 2001:12–18.

"Triglyceride, High-Density Lipoprotein and Coronary Heart Disease," NIH Consensus Panel on Triglyceride, High-density lipoprotein and coronary heart disease, *JAMA*, January 27, 1993; 269(4):505–510.

Accinni, R., Rosina, M., et al., "Effects of combined dietary supplementation on oxidative and inflammatory status in dyslipidemic subjects." *Nutr Metab Cardiovasc Dis*, 2006; 16(2):121-7.

Cleary, J.P., M.D., "Vitamin B3 in the treatment of diabetes mellitus: Case reports and review of the literature." *J Nutr Med*, 1990; 1:217-25.

Cunningham, John, J., Ph.D., "Micronutrients and nutraceutical interventions in diabetes mellitus," *Journal of the American College of Nutrition*, 1998; 17(1):7-10.

Elam, M.B., Hunninghake, D.B., Davis, K.B., et al., "Effect of niacin on lipid and lipoprotein levels and glycemic control in patients with diabetes and peripheral arterial disease. The ADMIT Study: A randomized trial." *JAMA*, September 13, 2000; 284(10):1263-1270.

Garg, A., Grundy, S.M., "Nicotinic acid as therapy for dyslipidemia in non-insulin-dependent diabetes mellitus." *JAMA*, 1990; 264(6):723-6.

Genest, Jacques, Jr., M.D., et al, "Prevalence of lipoprotein (a) [Lp(a)] excess in coronary artery disease." *American Journal of Cardiology*, 1991; 67:1039-1045.

Gosteli, J., "Nicotinamide trials in diabetes intervention: Does a metabolite provide benefit?" *Med Hypotheses*, 2005; 64(5):1062.

Hypponen, E., "Micronutrients and the risk of type 1 diabetes: Vitamin D, vitamin E, and nicotinamide." *Nutr Rev*, September 2004; 62(9):340–347.

Kaushik, S.V., Plaisance, E.P., et al., "Extended-release niacin decreases serum fetuin-A concentrations in individuals with metabolic syndrome." *Diabetes Metab Res Rev*, April 29, 2009.

Knip, M., Douek, I.F., Moore, W.P.T., et al., "Safety of high-dose nicotinamide: A review." *Diabetologia*, 2000; 43:1337–1345.

Manna, R., M.D., et al., "Nicotinamide treatment in subjects at high risk of developing insulin dependent diabetes improves insulin secretion." *British Journal of Clinical Practice*, Autumn 1992; 46(3):177–179.

Pociot, F., et al., "Nicotinamide - Biological actions and therapeutic potential in diabetes prevention, IDIG Workshop, Copenhagen, Denmark, 4–5 December 1992," *Diabetologia,* 1993; 36:574–576.

Pozzilli, P. et al., "Meta-analysis of nicotinamide treatment in patients with recent-onset IDDM. The Nicotinamide Trialists." *Diabetes Care,* 1996; 19(12):1357–63.

Pozzilli, B., et al, "Diabetes and nicotinamide, Nutrition Report, September 1995;59/double blind trial of nicotinamide in recent-onset insulin-dependent diabetes mellitus." *Diabetolog,* 1995; 38(7):848–852.

Pozzilli, Paolo, et al., "Vitamin E and nicotinamide have similar effects in maintaining residual beta cell function in recent onset insulin-dependent diabetes (the IMDIAB IV Study)." *European Journal of Endocrinology,* 1997; 137:234–239.

Pozzilli, Peak, et al., "Niacin aids remission of diabetes, The Nutrition Report." *Diabetalogia,* February 1989; 31:A533.

Wahlberg, G., et.al., "Protective effect of nicotinamide against nephropathy in diabetic rats." *Diabetes Res,* 1985; 2:307.

NICOTINIC ACID: THE ACID FORM OF VITAMIN B3

Canner, P.L., Furberg, C.D., et al., "Benefits of niacin in patients with versus without the metabolic syndrome and healed myocardial infarction (from the Coronary Drug Project)." *Am J Cardiol,* 2006; 97(4): 477–9.

Cashin-Hemphill, Linda, M.D., et al., "Beneficial effects of colestipol-niacin on coronary atherosclerosis: A four-year follow-up." *JAMA,* December 19, 1990; 264(23):3013–3017.

Knopp, R.H., *Am J Cardio,* 1998; 82.

Warnholtz, A., Wild, P., et al., "Effects of oral niacin on endothelial dysfunction in patients with coronary artery disease: results of the randomized, double-blind, placebo-controlled INEF study." *Atherosclerosis,* 2009; 204(1):216–21.

Zoler, M.L., "Niacin plus statin cuts coronary events by 70%." *Family Practice News,* January 1, 2001; 7.

VITAMIN B6

Coelingh Bennink, H.J.T., Schruers, W.H.P., "Improvement of oral glucose tolerance in gestational diabetes by pyridoxine." *Br Med J,* 1975; 3:13–15.

Cohen, K.L. et al., "Effect of pyridoxine (vitamin B6) on diabetic patients with peripheral neuropathy." *J Am Podiatry Assoc,* 1984; 74(8):394–7.

Folkers, K., "Evidence for a clinically significant deficiency of vitamin B6 in populations." *J Optimal Nutr,* 1993; 2(4):239–43.

Jones, C.L., Gonzales, V., "Pyridoxine deficiency: A new factor in diabetic neuropathy." *J AM Podiatry Assoc,* 1978; 68(9):646–53.

Levin, E.R., et al., "The influence of pyridoxine in diabetic peripheral neuropathy." *Diabetes Care,* 1981; 4 (6):606–9.

McCann, V.J., Davis, R.E., "Pyridoxine and diabetic neuropathy: a double-blind controlled study." Letter. *Diabetes Care,* 1983; 6(1):102–3.

McCann, V.J., Davis, R.E., "Serum pyridoxal concentrations in patients with diabetic neuropathy." *Aust N Z J Med,* 1978; 8:259–61.

Passariello, N. et al., "Effects of pyridoxine alpha-ketoglutarate on blood glucose and lactate in type I and type II diabetics." *Int J Clin.*

Rao, R.H., et al., "Failure of pyridoxine to improve glucose tolerance in diabetics." *J Clin Endocrinol Metab,* 1980; 50(1):198–200.

Ribaya-Mercado, J., et al., "Vitamin B6 deficiency elevates serum insulin in elderly subjects." *Ann N Y Acad Sci,* 1990; 585:531–3.

Rogers, K.S., Mohan, C., "Vitamin B6 metabolism and diabetes." *Biochem Med Metab Biol,* 1994; 52:10–17.

VITAMIN B12

"(Vitamin B12). A preliminary report." *Br J Ophthalmol,* 1958; 42:686–93.

Bhatt, H.R., et al., "Can faulty vitamin B12 (cobalamin) metabolism produce diabetic neuropathy? Letter to the Editor." *Lancet,* 1983; ii:572.

Cameron, A.J., Ahem, G.J., "Diabetic retinopathy and cyanocobalamin."

Ide, H., et al., "Clinical usefulness of intrathecal injection of methylcobalamin in patients with diabetic neuropathy." *Clin Ther,* 1987; 9(2):183–92.

Komerup, T., Strom, L., 'Vitamin B12 and retinopathy in juvenile diabetes.' *Acta Paediatr,* 1958; 47:646–51.

Sancetta, S.M., et al., "The use of vitamin B12 in the management of the neurological manifestations of diabetes mellitus, with notes on the administration of massive doses." *Ann Intern Med,* 1951; 35:1028–48.

Yaqub, B.A., et al., "Effects of methylcobalamin on diabetic neuropathy." *Clin Neurol Neurosurg,* 1992; 94(2):105–11.

BIOTIN

Coggeshall, J.C., et al., "Biotin status and plasma glucose in diabetics." *Ann N Y Acad Sci,* 1985; 447:389–92.

Koutsikos, D. et al., "Biotin for diabetic peripheral neuropathy." *Biomed Pharmacothe,* 1990; 44(10):511–14.

Maebashi, M., et al., "Therapeutic evaluation of the effect of biotin or hyperglycemia in patients with non-insulin dependent diabetes mellitus." *J Clin Biochem Nutr,* 1993; 14:211–18.

VITAMIN D

Jensen, T., et al., "Partial normalization by dietary cod-liver oil of increased microvascular albumin leakage in patients with insulin-dependent diabetes and albuminuria." *N Engl J Med,* 1989; 321:1572–7.

VITAMIN A

Basu, T.K., Basualdo, C.. "Vitamin A homeostasis and diabetes mellitus." *Nutrition,* 1997; 13(9):804–6.

Jensen, T. et al., "Partial normalization by dietary cod-liver oil of increased microvascular albumin leakage in patients with insulin-dependent diabetes and albuminuria." *N Engl J Med,* 1989; 321:1572–7.

Martinoli, L., et al., "Plasma retinol and alpha-tocopherol concentrations in insulin-dependent diabetes mellitus: their relationship to microvascular complications." *Int J Vitam Nutr Res*, 1993; 63(2):87–92.

THE VITAMIN E COMPLEX

Ayers, S., Jr., Mihan, R., "Vitamin E and dermatology." *Cutis*, 1975; 16:1017–21.

Beales, P.E., et al., "Vitamin E delays diabetes onset in the non-obese diabetic mouse." *Metab Res*, 1994; 26:450–2.

Block, M.T., "Vitamin E in the treatment of diseases of the skin." *Clin Med*, 1953; 60:31.

British Medical Journal, (cited in Bicknell & Prescott. The vitamins in medicine. Milwaukee: Lee Foundation, 1953, p 632) 1940; i 890.

Bursell, S.E., Clermont, A.C., Aiello, L.P., Aiello, L.M., Schlossman, D.K., Feener, E.P., Laffel, L., King, G.L., "High-dose vitamin E supplementation normalizes retinal blood flow and creatinine clearance in patients with type 1 diabetes." *Diabetes Care*, August 1999; 22(8):1245–51.

Devaraj, S., Jialal, I:, "Alpha tocopherol supplementation decreases serum C-reactive protein and monocyte interleukin-6 levels in normal volunteers and type 2 diabetic patients." *Free Radic Biol Med*, 2000; 29:790–2

Duntas, L., et al., "Administration of d-alpha tocopherol in patients with insulin-dependent diabetes mellitus." *Curr Ther Res*, 1996; 57:682–90.

Engelen, W., Keenoy, B.M., Vertommen, J., et al., "Effects of long-term supplementation with moderate pharmacologic doses of vitamin E are saturable and reversible in patients with type 1 diabetes." *Am J Clin Nutr*, 2000; 72:1142–9.

Fuller, C.J., et al., "R-(-tocopheryl acetate supplementation at pharmacologic doses decreases low-density-lipoprotein oxidative susceptibility but not protein glycation in patients with diabetes mellitus." *Am J Clin Nutr*, 1996; 63:753–9.

Gaede, P., Poulsen, H.E., Parving, H.H., et al., "Double-blind, randomized study of the effect of combined treatment with vitamin C and E on albuminuria in type 2 diabetic patients." *Diabet Med*, 2001; 18:756–60.

Gisinger, C., et al., "Vitamin E and platelet eicosanoids in diabetes mellitus." *Prostaglandins Leukot Essent Fatty Acids*. 1990; 40:169–76.

Granado, F.. et al., "Carotenoids, retinol and tocopherols in patients with insulin-dependent diabetes mellitus and their immediate relatives." *Clin Sci (Colch)*, 1998; 94(2):189–95.

Jain, S.K., et al., "The effects of modest vitamin E supplementation on lipid peroxidation products and other cardiovascular risk factors in diabetic patients." *Lipids*, 1996; 31(suppl):S87-S90.

Jain, S.K., et al., "Vitamin E (E) supplementation (placebo-controlled double-blind) lowers blood thromboxane and malondialdehyde (MDA) levels in type-1 diabetics (D). Abstract." *J AM Coll Nutr*, 1996; 15(5):536.

Koo, J.R., Ni, Z., Oviesi, F., Vaziri, N.D., "Antioxidant therapy potentiates antihypertensive action of insulin in diabetic rats." *Clin Exp Hypertens*, July 2002; 24(5):333–44.

Letter. *New England Journal of Medicine*, July 23, 1964; 271, 4.

Lubin, B., Machlin, L., "Biological aspects of vitamin E." *Ann N Y Acad Sci*, 1982; p. 393.

Luostarinin, R. et al., "Vitamin E supplementation counteracts the fish oil-induced increase of blood glucose in humans." *Nutr Res* 1995; 15:953–68.

Manzella, D., Barbieri, M., Ragno, E., et al., "Chronic administration of pharmacologic doses of vitamin E improves the cardiac autonomic nervous system in patients with type 2 diabetes." *Am J Clin Nutr*, 2001; 73:1052–7.

Martinoli, L., et al., "Plasma retinol and alpha-tocopherol concentrations in insulin-dependent diabetes mellitus: their relationship to microvascular complications." *Int J Vitam Nutr Res*, 1993; 63(2):87–92.

Paolisso, G., et al., "Daily vitamin E supplements improve metabolic control but not insulin secretion in elderly non-insulin-dependent diabetic patients." *Diabetes Care*, 1993; 16:1433–7.

Salonen, J.T., et al., "Increased risk of non-insulin diabetes mellitus at low plasma vitamin E concentrations: a four year follow-up study in men." *BMJ*, 1995; 311:1124–7.

Sano, M., Ernesto, C., Thomas, R.G., Klauber, M.R., Schafer, K., Grundman, M., Woodbury, P., Growdon, J., Cotman, C.W., Pfeiffer. E., Schneider, L.S., Thal, L.J., "A controlled trial of selegiline, alpha-tocopherol, or both as treatment for Alzheimer's disease. The Alzheimer's Disease Cooperative Study." *N Engl J Med*, April 24, 1997; 336(17):1216–22.

Shute, E., Shute, J.C.M.,(ed). *The Vitamin E Story*. Burlington, Ontario: Welch Publishing, 1985.

Skyrme-Jones, R.A., O'Brien, R.C., Berry, K.L., et al., "Vitamin E supplementation improves endothelial function in type 1 diabetes mellitus: a randomized, placebo-controlled study." *J Am Coll Cardiol*, 2000; 36:94–102.

Williams, H.T.G., Fenna, D., MacBeth, R.A., "Alpha tocopherol in the treatment of intermittent claudication." *Surgery, Gynecology and Obstetrics*, April 1971; 132:#4, 662–666.

THE FISH OILS

Das, U.N., et al., "Lipid peroxides and essential fatty acids in patients with diabetes mellitus and diabetic nephropathy." *J Nutr Med*, 1994; 4:149–55.

Friday, K.E., et al., "Omega-3 fatty acid supplementation has discordant effects on plasma glucose and lipoproteins in type II diabetes. Abstract." *Diabetes*, 1987; 36(Suppl 1):12A.

Glauber, H., et al., "Adverse metabolic effect of omega-3 fatty acids in non-insulin-dependent diabetes mellitus." *Ann Intem Med*, 1988; 108(5):663–8.

Kamada, T., et al., "Dietary sardine oil increases erythrocyte membrane fluidity in diabetic patients." *Diabetes*, 1986; 35:604–11.

McGrath, L.T., et al., "Effect of dietary fish oil supplementation of peroxidation of serum lipids in patients with non-insulin dependent diabetes mellitus." *Artherosclerosis*, 1996; 121:275–83.

McVeigh, G.E., et al., "Dietary fish oil augments nitric oxide production or release in patients with type 2 (non-insulin-dependent) diabetes mellitus." *Diabetologica*, 1993; 36(1):33–8.

Okuda, Y., et al., "Long-term effects of eicosapentaenoic acid on diabetic peripheral neuropathy and serum lipids in patients with type II and diabetes mellitus." *J Diabetic Complications*, 1996; 10:280–7.

Popp-Snijders, C., et al., "Dietary supplementation of omega-3 polyunsaturated fatty acids improves insulin sensitivity in non-insulin-dependent diabetes." *Diabetes Res*, 1987; 4:141–7.

Puhakainen, I., et al., "Dietary supplementation with n-3 fatty acids increases gluconeogenesis from glycerol but not hepatic glucose production in patients with non-insulin-dependent diabetes mellitus." *Am J Clin Nutr*, 1995; 61:121–6.

Vandongen, R., et al., "Hypercholesterolaemic effect of fish oil in insulin-dependent diabetic patients." *Med J Aust*, 1988; 148:141–3.

INOSITOL AND MYOINOSITOL

Clements, R.S., et al., "Dietary myo-inositol intake and peripheral nerve function in diabetic neuropathy." *Metabolism*, 1979; 28:477.

Gregersen, G., et al., "Myoinositol and function of peripheral nerves in human diabetics. A controlled clinical trial." *Acta Neurol Scand*, 1978; 58(4):241–8.

Gregersen, G., et al., "Oral supplementation of myoinositol: Effects on peripheral nerve function in human diabetics and on the concentration in plasma, erythrocytes, urine and muscle tissue in human diabetics and normals." *Acta Neurol Scand*, 1983; 67:164–72.

Mayhew, J.A., et al., "Free and lipid inositol, sorbitol and sugars in sciatic nerve obtained post-mortum from diabetic and control subjects." *Diabetologia*, 1983; 24:13–15.

Salway, J.G., et al., "Effect of myo-inositol on peripheral-nerve function in diabetes." *Lancet*, 1978; ii:1282.

Stevens, M.J., et al., "Acetyl-L-carnitine deficiency as a cause of altered nerve myo-inositol content, Na,K-ATPase activity, and motor conduction velocity in the streptozotocin-diabetic rat." *Metabolism*, 1996; 45(7):865–72.

CARNITINE

ALPHA LIPOIC ACID

Barbiroli, B., "Summarized in Conference Report: Thioctic acid - a rational remedy for the treatment of diabetic polyneuropathy." *Exp Clin Endocrinol Diabetes*, 1995; 104:126–7.

Jacob, S., et al., "Improvement of insulin-stimulated glucose-disposal in type 2 diabetes after repeated parenteral administration of thioctic acid." *Exp Clin Endocrinol Diabetes*, 1996; 104(3):284–8.

Lowitt, S., et al., "Acetyl-L-camitine corrects the altered peripheral nerve function of experimental diabetes." *Metabolism*, 1995; 44(5):677–80.

Quatraro, A., et al., "Acetyl-L-carnitine for symptomatic diabetic neuropathy." *Diabetalogica*, 1995; 38:123.

Stevens, M.J., et al., "Acetyl-L-carnitine deficiency as a cause of altered nerve myo-inositol content, Na,K-ATPase activity, and motor conduction velocity in the streptozotocin-diabetic rat." *Metabolism*, 1996; 45(7):865–72.

Ziegler, D., Gries, F.A., "A-lipoic acid in the treatment of diabetic peripheral and cardiac autonomic neuropath." *Diabetes*, 1997; 46(Suppl. 2):S62-S66.

Ziegler, D., Reljanovic, M., Mehnert, H., et al., "Alpha-lipoic acid in the treatment of diabetic polyneuropathy in Germany: current evidence from clinical trials." *Exp Clin Endocrinol Diabetes*, 1999; 107:421–30.

COENZYME Q10 AND Q7

Kishi, T., et al., "Bioenergetics in clinical medicine. IX. Studies on coenzyme Q and diabetes mellitus." *J Med*, 1976; 7:307.

Shigeta, Y., et al., "Effect of coenzyme Q7 treatment on blood sugar and ketone bodies of diabetics." *J Vitaminol*, 1966; 12:293.

EVENING PRIMROSE OIL

Haessler, H.A., Crawford, J.D., "Insulin-like inhibition of lipolysis and stimulation of lipogenesis by prostaglandin E1". *J Clin Invest*, 1967; 46:1065–70.

Houtsmuller, A.J., et al., "Favorable influences of linoleic acid on the progression of diabetic micro- and macroangiopathy." *Nutr Metab*, 1980; 24(Suppl 1):105–18.

Keen, H., et al., "Treatment of diabetic neuropathy with gamma-linolenic acid." *Diabetes Care*, 1993; 16(1):8–15.

Mercuri, O., et al., "Depression of microsomal desaturation of linoleic to gamma-linolenic acid in the alloxan-diabetic rat." *Biochim Biophys Acta*, 1966; 116:409–11.

FLAVONES

Gabor, M., "Pharmacologic effect of flavonoids on blood vessels." *Angiologica*, 1972; 9:355–74.

Magnard, G., et al., "Value of tetrahydroxy flavan-diol in ophthalmology, especially in chronic retinopathy (40 cases)." *Lyon Med*, 1970; 223(4):259–63 (in French).

Palmer, L.J., et al., "The influence of rutin upon diabetic retinitis." *Northwest Med*, 1951; 50:669–71.

Varma, S.D., et al., "Diabetic cataracts and flavonoids." *Science*, 1977; 195:205–6.

HERBAL MEDICINES IN DIABETES

Broadhurst, C.L., Polansky, M.M., Anderson, R.A., "Insulin-like biological activity of culinary and medicinal plant aqueous extracts in vitro." *J Agric Food Chem*, 2000; 48:849–52,

Kudolo, G.B., "The effect of 3-month ingestion of Gingo biloba extract (EGb 761) on pancreatic beta-cell function in response to glucose loading in individuals with non-insulin-dependent diabetes mellitus," *J Clin Pharmacol*, 2001; 41:600–11.

Pinn, G., "Herbs and metabolic/endocrine disease." *Aust Fam Physician*, 2000; 30:146–50.

Vogler, B.K., Ernst, E., "Aloe vera: a systematic review of its clinical effectiveness." *Br J Gen Pract*, 1999; 49:823–8.

PORTULACA

Andrade-Cetto, A., Heinrich, M., "Mexican plants with hypoglycemic effect used in the treatment of diabetes." *Journal of Ethnopharmacology*, 2005; 99(3): p325–348.

Rashed, N., F.U.A., Mayadeh, Shaedah, Taha A.M.O., "Investigation of the Active Constituents of Portulaca Asia Oleraceae L. (Portulacaceae) Growing In Jordan." *Pakistan Journal of Pharmaceutical Sciences*, 2004; Vol. 17(1):p.37–45.

Barbagallo, M., Dominguez, L.J., "Magnesium metabolism in type 2 diabetes mellitus, metabolic syndrome and insulin resistance." *Arch Biochem Biophys*, 2007; 458(1):40–7.

Braun, L.C., Cohen, M., "Herbs and Natural Supplements—An Evidence Based Guide." 2005.

Broadhurst, C.L., Domenico, P., "Clinical studies on chromium picolinate supplementation in diabetes mellitus—a review." *Diabetes Technol Ther,* 2006; 8(6):677–87.

Chiu, K.C., et al., "Hypovitaminosis D is associated with insulin resistance and beta cell dysfunction." *Am J Clin Nutr,* 2004; 79(5):820–5.

"Efficacy and safety of Purslane Herb Extract (PortusanaTM) in type II diabetic patients: a double-blind, placebo controlled clinical study in Frutarom corp independent data." Edith Wolfson Medical Center, Holon (Israel) 2006.

Dweck, A.C., "Purslane (Portulaca oleracea) - the global panacea." *Personal Care Magazine,* 2001; 2(4):7–15.

Gott, B., "Indigenous use of plants in south-eastern Australia." *Telopea,* 2008; 12(2):215–226.

Hassan-Wassef, H., "Food habits of the Egyptians: newly emerging trends." *La Revue de Santé de la Méditerranée orientale,* 2004; 10(6).

Kamil, M., Chan, K., Habibullah, M., "A review on Portulaca species -with special reference to Portulaca oleracea." *Aust J Med Herbalism,* 2000; 12(2).

Lai, M.H., "Antioxidant effects and insulin resistance improvement of chromium combined with vitamin C and e supplementation for type 2 diabetes mellitus." *J Clin Biochem Nutr,* 2008; 43(3):191–8.

Shen, "Effects of Portulaca Oleracea (Portusana TM) on Insulin Resistance in Rats with Type 2 Diabetes Mellitus." *Chinese J Med,* 2003; 9(4):289–292.

Simopoulos, A.P., "The Mediterranean Diets: What is so special about the diet of Greece? The scientific evidence." *J. Nutr,* 2001; 131(11):3065S–3073.

Viktorinova, A., et al., "Altered metabolism of copper, zinc, and magnesium is associated with increased levels of glycated hemoglobin in patients with diabetes mellitus." *Metabolism,* 2009.

Wang, H., Kruszewski, A., Brautigan, D.L., "Cellular chromium enhances activation of insulin receptor kinase." *Biochemistry,* 2005; 44(22):8167–75.

Yokota, K., "Diabetes mellitus and magnesium." *Clin Calcium,* 2005; 15(2):203–12.

GARLIC IN DIABETES

Adams, S.H., "Uncoupling protein homologs: emerging views of physiological function." *J Nutr,* 2000; 130(4):711–4.

Arsenault, B.J., et al., "Visceral adipose tissue accumulation, cardiorespiratory fitness, and features of the Metabol Forteic syndrome." *Arch Intern Med,* 2007; 167(14):1518–25.

Blumenthal, M., Goldberg, A., Brinckmann, J., ed. *Herbal Medicine - Expanded Commission E Monographs.* 2000, American Botanical Council.

Bordia, A., "Effect of garlic on blood lipids in patients with coronary heart disease." *Am J Clin Nutr,* 1981; 34(10):2100–3.

Bordia, A., Verma, S.K., Srivastava, K.C., "Effect of garlic (Allium sativum) on blood lipids, blood sugar, fibrinogen and fibrinolytic activity in patients with coronary artery disease." *Prostaglandins Leukot Essent Fatty Acids,* 1998; 58(4):257–63.

Bordia, A., Verma, S.K., Srivastava, K.C., "Effect of garlic on platelet aggregation in humans: a study in healthy subjects and patients with coronary artery disease." *Prostaglandins Leukot Essent Fatty Acids*, 1996; 55(3):201–5.

Braun, L., Cohen, M., *Herbs and Natural Supplements, An evidence-based guide.* 2005, Sydney: Elsevier Mosby.

Bulcao, C., et al., "The new adipose tissue and adipocytokines." *Curr Diabetes Rev*, 2006; 2(1):19–28.

Chan, K.C., Hsu, C.C., Yin, M.C., "Protective effect of three diallyl sulfides against glucose-induced erythrocyte and platelet oxidation, and ADP-induced platelet aggregation." *Thromb Res*, 2002; 108(5–6):317–22.

Cho, B.H., Xu, S., "Effects of allyl mercaptan and various allium-derived compounds on cholesterol synthesis and secretion in Hep-G2 cells." *Comp Biochem Physiol C Toxicol Pharmacol*, 2000; 126(2):195–201.

El-Demerdash, F.M., El-Naga, N.I., "Biochemical study on the hypoglycenic effects of onion and garlic in alloxan-induced diabetic rats." *Food Chem Toxicol*, 2005; 43:57–63.

ESCOP, Allii Sativi Monograph. Second Edition *European Scientific Cooperative On Phytotherapy; The Scientific Foundation For Herbal Medicinal Products.* 2003; Thieme.

Freedland, E.S., "Role of a critical visceral adipose tissue threshold (CVATT) in metabolic syndrome: implications for controlling dietary carbohydrates: a review." *Nutr Metab (Lond)*, 2004; 1(1):12.

Jain, R.C., Vyas, C.R., "Garlic in alloxan-induced diabetic rabbits." *Am J Clin Nutr*, 1975; 28(7):684–5.

Kang., S., "Decrement of adipocyte size and prevention of hyperlepinemia by garlic in high fat diet- induced obese rats." *Asia Pacific Journal of Clinical Nutrition*, 2005; (14)(Suppl).

Kojuri, J., Vosoughi, A.R., Akrami, M., "Effects of anethum graveolens and garlic on lipid profile in hyperlipidemic patients." *Lipids Health Dis*, 2007; 6:5.

Laclaustra, M., Corella, D., Ordovas, J.M., "Metabol Forteic syndrome pathophysiology: the role of adipose tissue." *Nutr Metab Cardiovasc Dis*, 2007; 17(2):125–39.

Liu, L. Yeh, Y.Y., "Inhibition of cholesterol biosynthesis by organosulfur compounds derived from garlic." *Lipids*, 2000; 35(2):197–203.

Nishimura, H., Higuchi, O., Tateshita, K., "Antioxidative activity of sulfur-containing compounds in Allium species for human LDL oxidation in vitro." *Biofactors*, 2004; 21(1–4):277–80.

O'Gara, E.A., Hill, D.J., Maslin, D.J., "Activities of garlic oil, garlic powder, and their diallyl constituents against Helicobacter pylori." *Appl Environ Microbiol*, 2000; 66(5):2269–73.

Ohta, R., et al., "In vitro inhibition of the growth of Helicobacter pylori by oil-macerated garlic constituents." *Antimicrob Agents Chemother*, 1999; 43(7):1811–2.

Oi, Y., et al., "Allyl-containing sulfides in garlic increase uncoupling protein content in brown adipose tissue, and noradrenaline and adrenaline secretion in rats." *J Nutr*, 1999; 129(2):336–42.

Qi, R., et al., "Inhibition by diallyl trisulfide, a garlic component, of intracellular Ca(2+) mobilization without affecting inositol-1,4, 5-trisphosphate (IP(3)) formation in activated platelets." *Biochem Pharmacol*, 2000; 60(10):1475–83.

Qureshi, A.A., et al., "Inhibition of cholesterol and fatty acid biosynthesis in liver enzymes and chicken hepatocytes by polar fractions of garlic." *Lipids,* 1983; 18(5):343–8.

Reaven, P., "Metabol Forteic syndrome." *J Insur Med,* 2004; 36(2):132–42.

Sendl, A., et al., "Inhibition of cholesterol synthesis in vitro by extracts and isolated compounds prepared from garlic and wild garlic." *Atherosclerosis,* 1992; 94(1):79–85.

Sheela, C.G., Kumud, K., Augusti, K.T., "Anti-diabetic effects of onion and garlic sulfoxide amino acids in rats." *Planta Med,* 1995; 61(4):356–7.

Venmadhi, S., D.T., "Studies on some liver enzymes in rats ingesting ethanol and treated with garlic oil." *Med. Sci. Res,* 1992; 20:729–731.

Wisneski, Leonard, A., M.D., "The Professional Reference to Conditions, Herbs and Supplements." *Integrative Medicine Communications Access 2000.*

Yeh, Y.Y., Liu, L., "Cholesterol-lowering effect of garlic extracts and organosulfur compounds: human and animal studies." *J Nutr,* 2001; 131(3s):989S–93S.

PERMEABLE CURCUMIN IN DIABETES

(ESCOP), *Curcumae Longae Rhizoma Monograph.* Second Edition Completely revised and expanded ed. European Scientific Cooperative On Phytotherapy. The Scientific Foundation For Herbal Medicinal Products 2003: Thieme

Ahmed, S., et al., "Biological basis for the Use of Botanicals in Osteoarthritis and Rheumatoid Arthritis: a review." *eCam,* 2005; 2(3):301–308.

Ammon, H., et al., "Mechanism of antiinflammatory actions of curcumine and boswellic acids." *J Ethnopharmacol,* 1993; 38(2–3):113–9.

Banerjee M, Tripathi, L.M., Srivastava, V.M., Puri, A., Shulka, R., "Modulation of inflammatory mediators by ibuprofen and curcumin treatment during chronic inflammation in rat." *Immunopharmacol. Immunotoxicol,* 2003; 25:213–224.

Barclay, L.R.C., et al., "On the Antioxidant Mechanism of Curcumin: Classical Methods Are Needed To Determine Antioxidant Mechanism and Activity." *Organic Letters,* 2000; 2(18):2841–2843.

Cao, W., et al., "Tumour necrosis factor-alpha up-regulates macrophage migration inhibitory factor expression in endometrial stromal cells via the nuclear transcription factor NF-kappaB." *Hum Reprod,* 2006; 21(2):421–8.

Chainani-Wu, N., "Safety and anti-inflammatory activity of curcumin: a component of tumeric (Curcuma longa)." *J Altern Complement Med,* 2003; 9(1):161–8.

Chopra, A., et al., Randomized double blind trial of an ayurvedic plant derived formulation for treatment of rheumatoid arthritis. *J Rheumatol,* 2000; 27(6):1365–72.

Conney, A.H., Lysz, T., Ferraro, T., Abidi, T.F., Manchand, P.S., Laskin, J.D., Huang, M.T., "Inhibitory effect of curcumin and some related dietary compounds on tumor promotion and arachidonic acid metabolism in mouse." *Adv. Enzyme Regul,* 1991; 31:385–396.

Deodhar, S.D., Sethi, R., Srimal, R.C., "Preliminary study on antirheumatic activity of curcumin (diferuloylmethane)." *Indian J. Med. Res,* 1980; 71:632–634.

ESCOP, *Curcumae Longae Rhizoma Monograph.* Second Edition ed. European Scientific Cooperative on Phytotherapy.

Funk, J.L.F., J. B. Oyarzo, J. N., et al., "Efficacy and mechanism of action of turmeric supplements in the treatment of experimental arthritis." *Arthritis Rheum*, 2006; 54(11): p. 3452–64.

Gaddipati, J.P., S.S., Calemine, J., Seth, P., Sidhu, G.S., Mahehwari, R.K., "(BioXtract ref 75) Differential regulation of cytokines and transcription factors in liver by curcumin following hemorrhage/resuscitation." *Shock*, 2003; 19:150–156.

Goel, A., B.C., Chauhan, D.P., "Specific inhibition of cyclooxygenase-2 (COX-2) expression by dietary curcumin in HT-29 human colon cancer cells." *Cancer Lett*, 2001; 172:111–118.

Kim, M., Choi, G., Lee, H., "Fungicidal property of Curcuma longa L. rhizome-derived curcumin against phytopathogenic fungi in a greenhouse." *J Agric Food Chem*, 2003; 51(6):1578–81.

Kohli, "Curcumin: A natural anti-inflammatory agent." *Indian L Pharmacol*, 2005; 37(3):141–147.

Lotz, M., "The role of nitric oxide in articular cartilage damage." *Rheum Dis Clin North Am*, 1999; 25(2):269–82.

Satoskar, R., Shah, S., Shenoy, S., "Evaluation of anti-inflammatory property of curcumin (diferuloyl methane) in patients with postoperative inflammation." *Int J Clin Pharmacol Ther Toxicol*, 1986; 24(12):651–4.

Srivastava, K.C., B.A., Verma, S.K., "Curcumin, a major component of food spice turmeric (Curcuma longa) inhibits aggregation and alters eicosanoid metabolism in human blood platelets." *Prostaglandins Leukot. Essent. Fatty Acids*, 1995; 52:223–227.

Steinert, A.F., et al., "Major biological obstacles for persistent cell-based regeneration of articular cartilage." *Arthritis Res Ther*, 2007; 9(3):213.

The Scientific Foundation For Herbal Medicinal Products, 2003; Thieme.

CINNAMON

Akilen, R., Robinson, N., et al., "Glycated hemoglobin and blood pressure-lowering effect of cinnamon in multi-ethnic Type 2 diabetic patients in the UK: a randomized, placebo-controlled, double-blind clinical trial." *Diabet Med*, 2010; 27(10):1159–67.

Crawford, P.J., "Effectiveness of cinnamon for lowering hemoglobin A1C in patients with type 2 diabetes: a randomized, controlled trial." *Am Board Fam Med*, 2009; 22(5):507–12.

Hlebowicz, J., Almer, L.O., et al., "Effect of cinnamon on postprandial blood glucose, gastric emptying, and satiety in healthy subjects." *Am J Clin Nutr*, 2007; 85(6):1552–6.

Hlebowicz, J., Hlebowicz, A., et al., "Effects of 1 and 3 g cinnamon on gastric emptying, satiety, and postprandial blood glucose, insulin, glucose-dependent insulinotropic polypeptide, glucagon-like peptide 1, and ghrelin concentrations in healthy subjects." *Am J Clin Nutr*, 2009; 89(3):815–21.

Kannappan, S., Jayaraman, T., et al., "Cinnamon bark extract improves glucose metabolism and lipid profile in the fructose-fed rat." *Singapore Med J*, 2006; 47(10):858–63.

Kirkham, S., Akilen, R., et al., "The potential of cinnamon to reduce blood glucose levels in patients with type 2 diabetes and insulin resistance." *Diabetes Obes Metab*, 2009; 11(12):1100–13.

Mang, B., Wolters, M., et al., "Effects of a cinnamon extract on plasma glucose, HbA, and serum lipids in diabetes mellitus type 2." *Eur J Clin Invest*, 2006; 36(5):340–4.

Preuss, H.G., Echard, B., et al., "Whole cinnamon and aqueous extracts ameliorate sucrose-induced blood pressure elevations in spontaneously hypertensive rats." *Journal of the American College of Nutrition,* 2006; 25(2):144–150.

Solomon, T.P., Blannin, A.K., et al., "Changes in glucose tolerance and insulin sensitivity following 2 weeks of daily cinnamon ingestion in healthy humans." *Eur J Appl Physiol,* 2009.

GYMNEMA SYLVESTRE

Al-Romaiyan, A., Liu, B., et al.,"A Novel Gymnema sylvestre extract stimulates insulin secretion from human islets in vivo and in vitro." *Phytotherapy Research,* 2010.

Walsh, N., "Asian herb for diabetes to be tested in clinical trial," *Family Practice News,* April 1, 2001; 22.

PANAX GINSENG

Vuksan, V., Sievenpiper, J.L., Koo, V.Y., et al., "American ginseng (Panax quinquefolius L) reduces postprandial glycemia in nondiabetic subjects and subjects with type 2 diabetes mellitus." *Arch Intern Med,* 2000; 160:1009–13.

Vuksan, V., Sung, M.K., et al., "Korean red ginseng (Panax ginseng) improves glucose and insulin regulation in well-controlled, type 2 diabetes: Results of a randomized, double-blind, placebo-controlled study of efficacy and safety." *Nutr Metab Cardiovasc Dis,* July 21, 2006.

AMINO ACIDS IN DIABETES: TAURINE AND SELENIUM

Allen, M.J., Lowry, R.W., "Successful reversal of retinitis pigmentosa." *Journal of Ortho-molecular Medicine,* 1998; 13(1):41–43.

Blaurock-Busch, E., Griffin, V., *Mineral and Trace Element Analysis,* 1996, TMI/MTM Books, Boulder, Colorado.

Florence, T.M., Setright, R.T., *The Handbook of Preventative Medicine,* 1994, Kingsclear Books, Crows Nest.

Clark, L.C., et al., "Decreased incidence of prostate cancer with selenium supplementation: results of a double-blind cancer prevention trial." *JAMA,* 1999; 2(1):14–18.

Heaney, A.P., et al., "Prevention of recurrent pancreatitis in familial lipoprotein lipase deficiency with high-dose anti-oxidant therapy." *J Clin Endocrinol Metab,* 84(4):1203–1205.

Yu, M.W., et al., Plasma selenium levels and risk of hepatocellular carcinoma among men with chronic hepatitis virus infection. *Am J Epidemiol,* 1999; 150(4):367–374.

Goodwin, J.K., Strickland, K.N., "The role of dietary modification and nondrug therapy in dogs and cats with congestive heart failure." *Vet Med,* October 1998; 919–926.

Hayes, K.C., et al., "Retinal degeneration associated with taurine deficiency in the cat." *Science,* 1975; 188:949–951.

Franconi, F., et al., "Plasma and platelet taurine are reduced in subjects with insulin-dependent diabetes mellitus: effects of taurine supplementation." *Am J Clin Nutr,* 1995; 61:1115–9.

Werbach, M.R., *Textbook of Clinical Nutritional Medicine,* 1999, Third Line Press, Inc, CA.

Clark, L.C., et al., "Effects of selenium supplementation for cancer prevention in patients with carcinoma of the skin; a randomized controlled trial." *JAMA*, 1996; 276(24): 1957–1962.

Bowery, D.J., et al., "Selenium deficiency and chronic pancreatitis: disease mechanism and potential for therapy." *HPB Surg*, 1999; 11(4):207–215.

Yoshizawa, K., et al., "Study of prediagnostic selenium level in toenails and the risk of advanced prostate cancer." *J Natl Cancer Inst*, 1998; 90:1219–1224.

Franconi, F., "Plasma and platelet taurine are reduced in subjects with insulin-dependent diabetes mellitus: effects of taurine supplementation." *Am. J Clin Nutr*, 1995; 61:1115–9.

Hyperhealth Health and Nutrition CD-Rom, Vol 99.1, In-Tele-Health, Vic.

Kirschmann, G.J., Kirschmann, J.D., 4th ed. *Nutrition Almanac*. 1996, McGraw Hill, New York.

Rea, W.J., *Chemical Sensitivity*, 1996, Vol 3. Lewis Publishers, New York.

Nakaya, Y., et al., "Taurine improves insulin sensitivity in the Otsuka Long-Evans Tokushima Fatty rat, a model of spontaneous type 2 diabetes." *Am. J Clin Nutr*, 2000; 71(1):54–58.

Editorial, "Dietary selenium: time to act." *BMJ*, 1997; 314:387.

Taylor, E.W., Nadimpalli, R.G., Ramanathan, C.S., "Genomic structures of viral agents in relation to the biosynthesis of selenoproteins." *Biol Trace Elem Res*; January 1997; 56(1):63–91.

Evans, M.E., Jones, D.P., Ziegler, T.R., "Glutamine inhibits cytokine-induced apoptosis in human colonic epithelial cells via the pyrimidine pathway." *Am J Physiol Gastrointest Liver Physiol*, 2005; 289(3):G388–96.

Schrauzer, G.N., "Nutritional selenium supplements: product types, quality, and safety." *J Am Coll Nutr*, 2001; 20(1):1–4.

Militante, J.D., Lombardini, J.B., "Treatment of hypertension with oral taurine: experimental and clinical studies." *Amino Acids*, 2002; 23(4):381–93.

Ciechanowska, B., 'Taurine as a regulator of fluid-electrolyte balance and arterial pressure." *Ann Acad Med Stetin*, 1997; 43:129–42.

Foos, T.M., Wu, J.Y., "The role of taurine in the central nervous system and the modulation of intracellular calcium homeostasis." *Neurochem Res*, 2002; 27(1–2):21–6.

Imaki, H., et al., "Retinal degeneration in 3-month-old rhesus monkey infants fed a taurine-free human infant formula." *J Neurosci Res*, 1987; 18:602–614.

Kulakowski, E.C., Maturo, J., "Hypoglycemic properties of taurine not mediated by enhance insulin release." *Biochem Pharmacol*, 1984; 33:2835–8.

May, S.W., Pollock, S.H., "Selenium-based anti-hypertensives: rationale and potential." *Drugs*, December 1998; 56(6):959–964.

Vinceti, M., et al., "Excess melanoma incidence in a cohort exposed to high levels of environmental selenium." *Cancer Epidemiol Biomarkers Prev*, October 1998;7:853–856.

Saito, Y., et al., (1998). "Effect of selenium deficiency on cardiac function of individuals with severe disabilities under long-term tube feeding." *Dev Med Child Neurol*, 1998; 40:743–748.

Yasushi, M., et al., "Is taurine effective for treatment of painful muscle cramps in liver cirrhosis?" *American Journal of Gastroenterology,* 1993; 88(9):1466–1467.

SAMe (S-Adenosyl Methionine)

Bottiglieri, T., "S-Adenosyl-L-methionine (SAMe): from the bench to the bedside—molecular basis of a pleiotrophic molecule." *Am. J. Clinical Nutrition,* 2002; 76(5):1151S–1157.

Braun, L., Cohen, M., *S-Adenosyl-L-Methionine, in Herbs and Natural Supplements. An evidence-based guide.* 2005, Elsevier Mosby Sydney. p. 321–5.

Gatto, G., et al., "Analgesizing effect of a methyl donor (S-adenosylmethionine) in migraine: an open clinical trial." *Int J Clin Pharmacol Res,* 1986; 6(1):15–7.

Grassetto, M., Varotto, A., "Primary fibromyalgia is responsive to S-adenosyl-L-methionine." *Current Therapeutic Research,* 1994; 55(7):797–806.

Lieber, C.S., Packer, L., "S-Adenosylmethionine: molecular, biological, and clinical aspects—an introduction." *Am J Clin Nutr,* 2002; 76(5):1148S–1150.

Lieber, C.S., "S-Adenosyl-L-methionine: its role in the treatment of liver disorders." *Am J Clin Nutr,* 2002; 76(5):1183S–1187.

Miller, A.L., "The methionine-homocysteine cycle and its effects on cognitive diseases." *Altern Med Rev,* 2003; 8(1):7–19.

Soeken, K.L., et al., "Safety and efficacy of S-adenosylmethionine (SAMe) for osteoarthritis: A meta-analysis." *J Fam Pract,* 2002; 51(5):425–30.

Stipanuk, M.H., *Homocysteine, Cysteine, and taurine, in Modern Nutrition in Health and Disease,* M.E. Shils, et al., Editors. 2005, Lippincott Williams & Wilkins: Baltimore, MD. p. 545–62.

ARGININE

Chowienczyk, P., Ritter, J., "Arginine: NO more than a simple amino acid?" *Lancet,* 1997; 250:901–2.

Lubec, B., et al., "L-arginine reduces lipid peroxidation in patients with diabetes mellitus." *Free Rad Biol Med,* 1997; 22(1–2):355–7.

Wascher, T.C., et al., "Effects of low-dose L-arginine on insulin-mediated vasodilation and insulin sensitivity." *Eur J Clin Invest,* 1997; 27:690–5.

METABOLIC SYNDROME

Christiansen, E., et al., "Intake of a diet high in trans monounsaturated fatty acids or saturated fatty acids. Effects on postprandial insulinemia and glycemia in obese patients with NIDDM." *Diabetes Care,* 1997; 20(5):881–7.

Kaplan, N.M., "The deadly quartet. Upper-body obesity, glucose intolerance, hypertriglyceridemia, and hypertension." *Arch Intern Med,* 1989; 149(7):1514–20.

Bulcao, C., et al., "The new adipose tissue and adipocytokines." *Curr Diabetes Rev,* 2006; 2(1):19–28.

Swade, T.F., Emanuele, N.V., "Alcohol & Diabetes." *Compr Ther,* 1997; 23(2):135–40.

Kelly, G.S., "Insulin resistance: lifestyle and nutritional interventions." *Altern Med Rev,* 2000; 5:109–132.

Thompson, D.H., Godin, D.V., "Micronutrients and antioxidants in the progression of diabetes." *Nutr Res,* 1995; 15:1377–410.

Freedland, E.S., "Role of a critical visceral adipose tissue threshold (CVATT) in metabolic syndrome: implications for controlling dietary carbohydrates: a review." *Nutr Metab* (Lond), 2004; 1(1):12.

Karam, J.H., et al., "The relationship of obesity and growth hormone to serum insulin levels." *Ann N Y Acad Sci*, 1965; 131(1):374–87.

Arsenault, B.J., et al., "Visceral adipose tissue accumulation, cardiorespiratory fitness, and features of the metabolic syndrome." *Arch Intern Med*, 2007; 167(14):1518–25.

Ford, E.S., Liu, S., "Glycemic index and serum high-density lipoprotein cholesterol concentration among us adults." *Arch Intern Med*, 2001; 161:572–6.

Murphy, K.G., Bloom, S.R., "Gut hormones in the control of appetite." *Exp Physiol*, 2004; 89(5):507–16.

Wren, A.M., Bloom,S.R., "Gut hormones and appetite control." *Gastroenterology*, 2007; 132(6):2116–30.

Steiner, G., "Editorial: From an excess of fat, diabetics die." *JAMA*, 1989; 262(3):398–9.

Laclaustra, Corella, D., Ordovas, J.M., "Metabolic syndrome pathophysiology: the role of adipose tissue." *Nutr Metab Cardiovasc Dis*, 2007; 17(2):125–39.

Obarzanek, E., Sacks, F.M., Vollmer, W.M., et al., "DASH Research Group. Effects on blood lipids of a blood pressure-lowering diet: the Dietary Approaches to Stop Hypertension (DASH) Trial." *Am J Clin Nutr*, 2001: 74:80–9.

Jenkins, D.J., et al., "Nibbling versus gorging: metabolic advantages of increased meal frequency." *N Engl J Med.* 1989; 321(14):929–34.

Bailey, C.J., "Treating insulin resistance: future prospects." *Diab Vasc Dis Res*, 2007; 4(1):20–31.

Wolever, T.M., et al., "The glycemic index: methodology and clinical implications." *Am J Clin Nutr,*1991; 54(5):846–54.

Brand-Miller, J., "Optimizing the cardiovascular outcomes of weight loss." *Am J Clin Nutr*, 2005; 81(5):949–50.

Mustard, J.F., Packam, M.A., "Platelets and diabetes mellitus." *N Engl J Med*, 1994; 311:665–7.

McMillan-Price, J., et al., "Comparison of 4 diets of varying glycemic load on weight loss and cardiovascular risk reduction in overweight and obese young adults: a randomized controlled trial." *Arch Intern Med*, 2006; 166(14):1466–75.

Jenkins, D.J., et al., "Metabolic advantages of spreading the nutrient load: effects of increased meal frequency in non-insulin-dependent diabetes." *Am J Clin Nutr*, 1992; 55:461–7.

Kuo, L.E., et al., "Neuropeptide Y acts directly in the periphery on fat tissue and mediates stress-induced obesity and metabolic syndrome." *Nat Med*, 2007; 13(7):803–11.

Sarabi, M., Lind, L., "Mental stress opposes endothelium-dependent vasodilation in young healthy individuals." *Vasc Med*, 2001; 6(1):3–7.

Liu, S., Manson, J.E., Stampfer, M.J., et al., "Dietary glycemic load assessed by food-frequency questionnaire in relation to plasma high-density-lipoprotein cholesterol and fasting plasma triacylglycerols in postmenopausal women." *Am J Clin Nutr*, 2001; 73:560–6.

Spreitsma, J.E., Schuitemaker, G.E., "Diabetes can be prevented by reducing insulin production." *Med Hypotheses*, 1994; 42(1):15–23.

Stoney, C.M., et al., "Acute psychological stress reduces plasma triglyceride clearance." *Psychophysiology*, 2002; 39(1):80–5.

Brighthope, I., ACNEM lectures 2007.

Spiegel, K., et al., "Brief communication: Sleep curtailment in healthy young men is associated with decreased leptin levels, elevated ghrelin levels, and increased hunger and appetite.' *Ann Intern Med*, 2004; 141(11):846–50.

Taheri, S., et al., "Short sleep duration is associated with reduced leptin, elevated ghrelin, and increased body mass index." *PLoS Med*, 2004; 1(3):e62.

Schardt, D., "How sleep affects your weight." *Nutrition Action Healthletter*, July-August 2005.

SUGAR, OBESITY AND HEART DISEASE

Welsh, J.A., Sharma, A., Cunningham, S.A., Vos, M.B., "Consumption of added sugars and indicators of cardiovascular disease risk among US adolescents." *Circulation*, January 25, 2011; 123(3):249–57, Epub January 10, 2011.

EXERCISE: I LOVE WALKING IN THE PARK

Dwyer, T., et al., "Association of change in daily step count over five years with insulin sensitivity and adiposity: population based cohort study" *BMJ*, 2011; 342:c7249.

INDEX